AF840555

Education in a Competitive and Globalizing World Series

NEW RESEARCH IN EDUCATION: ADULT, MEDICAL AND VOCATIONAL

EDUCATION IN A COMPETITIVE AND GLOBALIZING WORLD SERIES

Motivation in Education
Desmond H. Elsworth (Editor)
2009. ISBN: 978-1-60692-234-7

The Reading Literacy of U.S. Fourth-Grade Students in an International Context
Justin Baer, Stéphane Baldi, Kaylin Ayotte,Patricia J. Gree and Daniel McGrath
2009 ISBN: 978-1-60692-138-3

Teacher Qualificationsand Kindergartners' Achievements
Cassandra M. Guarino, Laura S. Hamilton, J.R. Lockwood,Amy H. Rathbun and Elvira Germino Hausken
2009 ISBN: 978-1-60741-180-2

Effects of Family Literacy Interventions on Children's Acquisition of Reading
Ana Carolina Pena (Editor)
2009 ISBN: 978-1-60741-236-6

Nutrition Education and Change
Beatra F. Realine (Editor)
2009. ISBN: 978-1-60692-983-4

Reading at Risk: A Survey of Literary Reading in America
Rainer D. Ivanov
2009. ISBN: 978-1-60692-582-9

Evaluating Online Learning: Challenges and Strategies for Success
Arthur T. Weston (Editor)
2009. ISBN: 978-1-60741-107-9

Learning in the Network Society and the Digitized School
Rune Krumsvik (Editor)
2009. ISBN: 978-1-60741-172-7

Rural Education in the 21st Century
Christine M.E. Frisiras (Editor)
2009 ISBN: 978-1-60692-966-7

IT- Based Project Change Management System
Faisal Manzoor Arain
2009. ISBN: 978-1-60741-148-2

Reading: Assessment, Comprehensionand Teaching
Nancy H. Salas and Donna D. Peyton
2009 ISBN: 978-1-60692-615-4

Mentoring: Program Development, Relationships and Outcomes
Michael I. Keel (Editor)
2009. ISBN: 978-1-60692-287-3

Enhancing Prospects of Longer-Term Sustainability of Cross-Cultural INSET Initiatives in China
Chunmei Yan
2009. ISBN: 978-1-60741-615-9

Multimedia in Education and Special Education
Onan Demir and Cari Celik
2009. ISBN 978-1-60741-073-7

PCK and Teaching Innovations
Syh-Jong Jang
2009. ISBN: 978-1-60741-147-5

Academic Administration: A Quest for Better Management and Leadership in Higher Education
Sheying Chen (Editor)
2009. ISBN: 978-1-60741-732-3

Reading: Assessment, Comprehension and Teaching
Nancy H. Salas and Donna D. Peyton (Editors)
2009. ISBN: 978-1-60876-543-0

New Research in Education: Adult, Medical and Vocational
Edmondo Balistrieri and Giustino DeNino (Editors)
2009. ISBN: 978-1-60741-873-3

Education in a Competitive and Globalizing World Series

NEW RESEARCH IN EDUCATION: ADULT, MEDICAL AND VOCATIONAL

EDMONDO BALISTRIERI
AND
GIUSTINO DENINO
EDITORS

Nova Science Publishers, Inc.
New York

Copyright © 2009 by Nova Science Publishers, Inc.

All rights reserved. No part of this book may be reproduced, stored in a retrieval system or transmitted in any form or by any means: electronic, electrostatic, magnetic, tape, mechanical photocopying, recording or otherwise without the written permission of the Publisher.

For permission to use material from this book please contact us:
Telephone 631-231-7269; Fax 631-231-8175
Web Site: http://www.novapublishers.com

NOTICE TO THE READER

The Publisher has taken reasonable care in the preparation of this book, but makes no expressed or implied warranty of any kind and assumes no responsibility for any errors or omissions. No liability is assumed for incidental or consequential damages in connection with or arising out of information contained in this book. The Publisher shall not be liable for any special, consequential, or exemplary damages resulting, in whole or in part, from the readers' use of, or reliance upon, this material. Any parts of this book based on government reports are so indicated and copyright is claimed for those parts to the extent applicable to compilations of such works.

Independent verification should be sought for any data, advice or recommendations contained in this book. In addition, no responsibility is assumed by the publisher for any injury and/or damage to persons or property arising from any methods, products, instructions, ideas or otherwise contained in this publication.

This publication is designed to provide accurate and authoritative information with regard to the subject matter covered herein. It is sold with the clear understanding that the Publisher is not engaged in rendering legal or any other professional services. If legal or any other expert assistance is required, the services of a competent person should be sought. FROM A DECLARATION OF PARTICIPANTS JOINTLY ADOPTED BY A COMMITTEE OF THE AMERICAN BAR ASSOCIATION AND A COMMITTEE OF PUBLISHERS.

LIBRARY OF CONGRESS CATALOGING-IN-PUBLICATION DATA

New research in education : adult, medical, and vocational / [edited by] Edmondo Balistrieri and Giustino DeNino.
p. cm.
Includes index.
ISBN 978-1-60741-873-3 (hardcover)
1. Adult education. 2. Medical education. 3. Vocational education. I. Balistrieri, Edmondo. II. DeNino, Giustino.
LC5215.N468 2009
374--dc22

2009021728

Published by Nova Science Publishers, Inc. ✦ New York

CONTENTS

PREFACE

In a broad sense, education refers to any act or experience that has a formative effect on the mind, character, or physical ability of an individual. Adult education has become common in many countries. It takes on many forms, ranging from formal class-based learning to self-directed learning. It often takes place in the workplace, at secondary schools or at a college or university level. Similarly, vocational education prepares learners for jobs that are based in manual or practical activities. Vocational education can also be at the secondary or post-secondary level. Alternatively, medical education refers to the education related to the practice of being a medical practitioner. Medical education and training varies considerably across the world. This book reviews the most current research done on these topics from around the globe.

Chapter 1 - This paper uses micro-data from the University of Western Australia Graduate Destination Survey, linked to information from the University's Student Records System, to explore the determinants of students' academic performance at university and their starting salaries upon graduation. While the study also examines the impacts of gender, birthplace, prior academic achievement, and high school attended, most emphasis is placed on the impacts of age and field of study. The special emphasis on age enables conclusions to be drawn on whether mature-aged students can compete with younger adults, both in terms of academic success and success in the labor market. The findings of the research should have relevance to the development of transitional programs for adults entering university, and the design of study programs that might be best suited to their life stag China's adult and continuing education has undergone dramatic changes in recent years following the rapid expansion of enrollment in universities. This article examines strategies and approaches that adult and continuing education in China has responded to the challenges and opportunities. It first attempts to provide a critical review of neoliberal policies of marketization in higher education. Then historical perspectives of adult and continuing education in China are given, and this analysis is aimed at contributing to a better understanding of the development of China's adult and continuing education sector. Following this review, the strategies of responses are explored in detail to examine how the restructuring has impacted on the adult higher education system and institutional structure, which in turn will decide whether educators in adult and continuing education can efficiently address the relevant needs in this changing economic and social environment and provide the high quality of professional continuing education programs. It concludes that the strategies adopted by adult and continuing education in China have been consistent with the global trend of marketization in higher education.

Chapter -2 - China's adult and continuing education has undergone dramatic changes in recent years following the rapid expansion of enrollment in universities. This article examines strategies and approaches that adult and continuing education in China has responded to the challenges and opportunities. It first attempts to provide a critical review of neoliberal policies of marketization in higher education. Then historical perspectives of adult and continuing education in China are given, and this analysis is aimed at contributing to a better understanding of the development of China's adult and continuing education sector. Following this review, the strategies of responses are explored in detail to examine how the restructuring has impacted on the adult higher education system and institutional structure, which in turn will decide whether educators in adult and continuing education can efficiently address the relevant needs in this changing economic and social environment and provide the high quality of professional continuing education programs. It concludes that the strategies adopted by adult and continuing education in China have been consistent with the global trend of marketization in higher education.

Chapter 3 - Sir William Osler, the 'Father of Modern Medicine,' said "If you listen carefully to the patient, he will tell you the diagnosis." Today, physicians face increasing pressure to expedite medical care, often to the detriment of fully listening to the patient. Consequently, physicians use written screening tools to save time and theoretically facilitate communication with the patient. Physicians hope that patients will generate the diagnosis themselves, a 21st century compromise between modern time constraints and Oslerian communication and observation.

However, what if a patient administers a questionnaire inaccurately? The authors have shown that up to 70% of patients misrepresent their symptoms on common written screening tools. Given the role of screening tools in place of part of the medical interview, these inaccurate scores could influence medical decisions, placing patients with low health literacy at increased risk for inappropriate management, such as unnecessary surgery. Consequently, the authors designed an electronic screening tool that reduces misunderstanding and improves patient satisfaction. Through this novel use of technology, they have reconciled screening tools with Osler's concept of communication and observation. As a result, patients in our clinic are safer, better managed, and more satisfied.

Chapter 4 - The paper explores the promise, problems and pitfalls of vocational forms of secondary schooling when these are set up in developing countries. Taking Ghana as a case study, the author presents empirical evidence to examine some of the assumptions of human capital theory, and concludes that there are important limitations which prevent vocational schools from responding adequately to the requirements for economic development. The reasons for the failure of such innovations need to be identified not only from within the educational institution, but also from the wider macro-economic perspective.

Chapter 5 - There is a demand for more flexible delivery approaches in Vocational Education and Training, which has led to greater exploration of the use of Information and Communications Technology (ICT). This chapter describes a collaborative approach used by a small team of trade teachers seeking to develop ICT resources to help meet the requirements of their Registered Training Organization (RTO). The institutional policy of the RTO is shifting to favor a constructivist, project-based, approach to learning over traditional instructional pedagogy, as well as industry and individual requirements for more flexible learning options.

Chapter 6 - The "voice" of students with disabilities typically goes unheard. Valuable insights to strengthen academic and social learning are missed when students are not consulted with or listened to. This chapter describes the use of graphic facilitation to capture the voice of a group of four young adults with special educational needs. Participation in a conference presentation enabled them to share personal ideas about their secondary school experiences with a group of special educators. The special educators who observed the process found that it was an effective way to hear and capture the student voice. It provided them with valuable insights and information for the ongoing development of the meaningful and supportive educational programmes in secondary schools. Listening to the voice of young people and involving them in the design of the educational experience will turn up the volume to ensure that the voice fashions the educational journey.

Chapter 7 - Learner study guides are increasingly used in health professions' curricula. Their importance lies in their explicitness about what is to be taught and learned and their ability to identify the core. They are a key tool in the promotion of self-directed learning and tell the learners what to learn; how to learn it; and whether they have learned it.

Study guides have three roles: provision of content; management of learning; and student activities. Two models for study guide development are provided: TOPICAL for clinical courses; and TRACKER for distance learning. Convenience, language and readability, instructional design, and format need consideration when preparing a study guide.

The advantages of study guides include the ability to support the educational strategies of the institution and making education more effective. Potential disadvantages include: being too prescriptive and 'spoon-feeding'; queries about suitability for all learning styles; the teacher time involved in the development; being resource intensive; and the need for regular updating. These disadvantages, however, can be overcome in practice and are out weighed by the advantages. A model for the key features of study guides "the ten Is" is presented.

Chapter 8 - The apprenticeship model for teaching tha art and science medicine has long been the mainstay of graduate medical education (GME). Significant change in the health care environment however has resulted in a new set of challenges and growing public and private calls for reform in the GME process. In response to these calls, there has been an emerging consensus to move from the traditional "apprenticeship model" to a new "competency model" of education. External and internal stakeholders in the health care system (e.g., regulatory agencies, private nongovernmental professional organizations, insurance companies, industry, and the public) now demand "proof of quality" based upon evidence, external measures of performance, data driven improvements, and quantifiable outcomes. Due in part to these external pressures new competencies have emerged for GME that will require the development of new tools to both teach and assess "competence" in the "competencies". The Accreditation Council for Graduate Medical Education (ACGME) in the United States has proposed six specific new competencies including patient care, medical knowledge, communication and interpersonal skills, professionalism, practice based learning, and systems based practice.

This short communication will describe the six ACGME competencies, the emerging tools that might be used to both teach and assess these competencies; the current concepts and educational models guiding tool development and testing, and the results of an implementation process in the field of ophthalmology. The new ACGME competencies will require the development and testing of specific tools that will form the basis of a competency toolbox. These tools ideally would include both formative and summative feedback, faculty oversight, structured learning activities, specific scoring rubrics with behavioral anchors, benchmark and aggregate data, and linkage to improved downstream patient outcomes (e.g., quality, medical error reduction, patient safety, cost effectiveness). The barriers to implementation as well as examples of small successes and progress will be described. The challenge for organized medicine is developing an integrated, systematic, reliable and valid approach for GME to move from the "apprenticeship model" towards a "competency based" model.

Chapter 9 - This chapter asserts that "there is nothing more practical than a good theory", and. as professional practice is better understood, theory will both inform practice and to be informed by it. Already, a body of theory has accumulated which can inform practice, and the author shows this by reviewing conclusions drawn from his earlier monograph on the application of eight educational theories to medical education. This is followed by a discussion of three different theories: cognitive apprenticeship, multiple intelligences, , and conditions of learning. A brief overview is provided of each of these theories followed by a discussion of their implications for educational practice., including a specific example for each drawn from medical education.

Chapter 10 - Medical schools should devote more time and energy to helping medical students improve their decision making skills. Such instruction should include, at a minimum, an introduction to the theory of rational choice, an outline of the empirical research on human irrationality, and familiarisation with some of the tools and techniques that have been developed to help people to behave more rationally, such as decision-support systems and cognitive forcing strategies. The first and most important means for helping medical students to make more rational decisions is to introduce them to the research on cognitive biases, and to encourage them to analyse their own behaviour in the light of this research.

In: New Research in Education Adult, Medical and Vocational ISBN 978-1-60741-873-3
Editors: Edmondo Balistrieri and Giustino DeNino © 2009 Nova Science Publishers, Inc.

Chapter 1

ACADEMIC PERFORMANCE AND GRADUATE OUTCOMES: DOES AGE MATTER?*

Ian Li and Paul W. Miller
Business School
The University of Western Australia, Perth, Australia

ABSTRACT

This paper uses micro-data from the University of Western Australia Graduate Destination Survey, linked to information from the University's Student Records System, to explore the determinants of students' academic performance at university and their starting salaries upon graduation. While the study also examines the impacts of gender, birthplace, prior academic achievement, and high school attended, most emphasis is placed on the impacts of age and field of study. The special emphasis on age enables conclusions to be drawn on whether mature-aged students can compete with younger adults, both in terms of academic success and success in the labor market. The findings of the research should have relevance to the development of transitional programs for adults entering university, and the design of study programs that might be best suited to their life stage.

I. INTRODUCTION

Education is important to the individual, and to society as a whole. In terms of the individual, "…a man qualifies himself for occupational life by obtaining an education; as a consequence of pursuing his occupation, he obtains income" (Duncan, 1961, p.116). Education, therefore, is promoted as the key to an individual's economic success. From society's perspective, "The nation's prospects will be determined by the efficient and effective use of all its resources—particularly its human resources…to do this the higher

* Miller acknowledges financial support from the Australian Research Council. Views in this paper are those of the authors, and should not be attributed to the University of Western Australia or Graduate Careers Australia.

education sector and the vocational education and training sector must find effective ways to work together to produce the knowledge and skills that the nation requires" (Department of Education, Employment and Workplace Relations (DEEWR), 2008, p.4). One of the ways that the higher education sector in Australia is expected to develop is through providing opportunities for older adults to upgrade and refresh their skills (DEEWR, 2008, p.21).

Older adults have always had a major presence in the tertiary student population in Australia. For example, in 1980 students aged 25 or more years accounted for 39 percent of the 322,964 students in higher education.[1] In 1990 they accounted for 38 percent of the 485,866 higher education students. By 2007 the higher education student population had grown to 1,029,846 students, and 390,602, or 38 percent, of these were aged 25 or more years. These mature-age students are the focus of this study.

The structure of the paper is as follows. Section II presents a brief review of the literature on differences in academic and graduate labor market outcomes on the basis of age. Section III introduces the data used in the empirical section of this study, and outlines how these data can be utilized to study academic outcomes and graduate labor market outcomes. Section IV presents the findings from the empirical investigations. Section V concludes with a summary and policy recommendations.

II. Age and Academic and Labor Makret Success: What Do We Already Know?

(A) Age and Academic Success

There is a rather extensive literature examining the impact of age on academic performance. Most of the studies to date, however, have been focussed on early learning outcomes or students of a young age rather than on higher education students, which are the focus of this study. It is, nevertheless, instructive to review the evidence from these studies based on younger students, as some of the factors that affect academic outcomes at an early age may persist over time (see, for example, Goodman and Sianesi, 2005), and, to the extent that this is the case, studies of younger children will be able to inform the current study of university students' academic performance. Moreover, the most relevant studies on higher education students have been largely descriptive, and have reported mixed findings on the relationships between age and academic outcomes, and study of the literature on early childhood achievement may assist our understanding of the reasons for this.

Studies of age effects on early childhood outcomes have often differentiated between three groups of students: students who have entered school at the conventional age and have progressed normally through the school grades; students who entered school at the conventional age but have repeated at least one grade; and students whose entry into the school system was delayed intentionally. The latter practice is motivated by arguments that older students in a school grade have higher levels of academic achievement and/or are socially and emotionally better equipped to deal with life at school. The emphasis given to the

[1] The data in this paragraph are from the DEEWR website (DEEWR, 2009).

alternative arguments for the age effects on early school achievements varies across studies, however, with some focussing on the links between older students' better academic performance and their relative maturity (for example, see Del Bono and Galindo-Rueda, 2004) and others on the theorized superior cognitive skills of older students (for example, see Datar, 2006).

Many studies report evidence of favorable age effects on early school achievements. Langer *et al.* (1984), for example, report that older students have superior achievement scores (based on reading, mathematics and sciences exercises), and are also less likely to repeat classes. However, these effects are stronger in samples covering earlier school grades than they are in samples covering later school grades. Likewise, Goodman and Sianesi (2005) found that older students were associated with superior academic outcomes, and while this advantage appeared to diminish over time, the academic advantage remained up until age 16. The findings in Stipek and Byler's (2001) study, based on longitudinal data, are similar.

This general pattern in the age effects on the academic achievements of school-aged children appears to carry over to more comprehensive, cross-national studies. For instance, Bedard and Dhuey (2006) examined the academic outcomes of students across different OECD countries and find that the oldest students score 4 to 12 percent higher than their youngest peers in the fourth grade.[2] Similarly, the oldest students in the eighth grade[3] score 2 to 9 percent higher than their youngest peers. Bedard and Dhuey (2006) also widen the range of age effects examined. They report that relatively older students are more likely to participate in core-university academic programs during the final years of high school, and also are more likely to attend a good postsecondary institution.[4]

However, some of the age effects reported are inconsistent with delayed entry being beneficial to a student's academic outcomes. Byrd *et al.* (1997), for example, reported adverse behavioral consequences for older students, regardless of whether they were repeat-students or had delayed entry. To the extent that these behavioral problems impact academic achievements, it would be expected that older students would perform less well at school than their younger counterparts. Evidence along these lines is found in the study by Graue and DiPerna (2000), where repeat-students and students with delayed entry are shown to under-perform compared to students who commenced school at the conventional age and who did not repeat any classes. Of the two groups of older students, the repeat-students fared worse than the delayed entry students. May *et al.* (1995) found that students who were older when they commenced school were more likely to access special needs education. However, there was no significant effect of delayed entry on grade progression.

Thus, the literature on relative age effects among school children generally finds that older students have better academic outcomes as a result of their relative maturity, or due to their more advanced cognitive skills, though studies with the opposite findings make for a somewhat muddy overall assessment. Much of the evidence suggests that the age effects dissipate as higher grades are examined, and thus it might be expected that any age effects among university students would be quite weak.

---

[2] The typical age of a student in the fourth grade is 9 to 10 years old.

[3] Eighth graders are typically 13 to 14 years old.

[4] Fredriksson and Ockert (2005) also widen the ambit of the age factor to consider the effects for particular subjects. They report that older students achieved better academic outcomes in all subjects.

Given the findings on age effects on early childhood achievements, it is not surprising that mixed findings have been reported on the role that age might have on tertiary academic performance. As summarised by Birch and Miller (2008) in relation to the research in Australia, "Some studies report that younger students perform better at university than older students (e.g., Long *et al.*, 1994), others find the opposite (e.g., Smyth *et al.*, 1990 and Cantwell *et al.*, 2001), while some even find that students' tertiary academic performance is not influenced by their age (e.g., Dickson *et al.*, 2000 and McKenzie and Schweitzer, 2001). Birch and Miller (2008) report positive relationships between age and academic performance in the first year of university study, between age and the probability of students continuing with their university studies beyond the first year, and between age and academic performance in the second and third years of study, although these effects were typically quite small.

(B) Age and Graduate Starting Salaries

Age may be related to the earnings of individuals with a given educational attainment for the same sort of reasons noted in the literature on academic performance. Specifically, to the extent that for a given level of schooling, age is associated with greater maturity and social development and cognitive ability, then it would be expected to lead to higher wages. However, as the literature on age effects on academic performance reviewed above suggests that these effects are weaker among secondary school students than among primary school students (see, for example, Goodman and Sianesi, 2005), the age effects on labor market outcomes that derive from these sources may be quite weak.

A further factor that is associated with age in the literature on academic performance is behavioral problems (see Byrd *et al*,, 1997). These may also impact labor market outcomes. Le *et al.* (2005) show that individuals who experience conduct disorder problems at an early age are more likely to leave school early, have poorer employment prospects and lower earnings.

However, when the focus is on mature-age students, the age variable may largely capture prior labor market experience, or general skills acquired through learning-by-living. This is the interpretation placed on the age variable in the recent studies of graduate starting salaries in Australia by Chia and Miller (2008) and Birch, Li and Miller (2009).

Klevmarken and Quigley (1976) formalize these arguments, though the learning effects they theorise are contrary to those established in many of the studies of early childhood academic outcomes. Thus, they consider three groups in a graduation cohort: the first are those who are younger than is typical of the cohort (termed "quick" by the authors); the second are those who are of the usual or typical age ("normal"); and the third are those who are older ("slow"). Klevmarken and Quigley (1976, p.30) argued, "The 'quick' group is made up of students who are more efficient in learning than average but who graduate with no previous labor market experience; the 'normal' group contains students of average ability who graduate with no (or very little) previous labor market experience; and the 'slow' group contains those who are perhaps less efficient in learning than average but are often those with additional labor market experience. In general, one would expect that students who are efficient in learning are also efficient in productive work. For this reason, their potential starting salaries would tend to be high. However, previous labor market experience would also increase their potential starting salaries". Klevmarken and Quigley (1976, p.65) thus argue that there will be a U-shaped relationship between starting salary and age, with this being driven by the greater ability of the relatively young 'quick' group, and the greater labor market experience of the relatively old 'slow' group. In analyses that control for academic performance at university, however, it would be expected that the latter influence will dominate, and there will be a positive relationship between age and starting salary.

Thus, the literature suggests that while there may be age effects on academic performance at university, these are likely to be modest. Stronger, positive age effects are expected in the analysis of graduates' starting salaries in the encompassing models proposed below that include controls for academic achievement.

III. Data and Estimating Equations

The data used in this study are from Chia and Miller (2008). They analysed a data set that combined information from a survey of the labor market (and other) destinations of graduates (termed the Graduate Destination Survey) with details on those graduates from the Student Records System at the University of Western Australia. These data cover graduates who received a bachelor's degree from the University between 2002 and 2004. Full details are presented in Chia and Miller (2008), and only summary comments are provided here.

The Graduate Destination Survey (GDS) is part of a national data collection program that aims to take a snapshot of the activities of recent graduates around four months after they completed their degree (Graduate Careers Australia, 2009). While the surveys are organised by Graduate Careers Australia, they are conducted through each of the universities in Australia. Given this way of running the survey out of each university, it is possible to merge the information collected by a particular university with the information that university has on each student's academic profile, including demographic characteristics, course enrolment, and academic achievements.[5] This is what Chia and Miller (2008) did for the University of Western Australia.

The analyses in Chia and Miller (2008) and the current study are restricted to graduates who completed a bachelor's degree and who have valid starting salary data and information on other characteristics included in the statistical analyses that follow. Further, only domestic students who replied to the survey were included in the analysis. The sample size is 2143.

The information available for analysis includes academic achievement at university and at high school, field of study, degree type, course type, attendance type, data on the high school attended, students' demographic characteristics, including age, gender, birthplace and the year of arrival in Australia among the foreign born, annual starting salaries, hours worked per week, sector of employment, employment type, study status, and occupation. Full details are presented in Appendix A.

These data are used to estimate two models: a model of tertiary academic achievement and a model of graduate starting salaries. Chia and Miller (2008) did not examine tertiary

---

[5] All graduates are approached to complete the survey, but the response rate at the University of Western Australia is only around 50 percent. A detailed examination of the non-respondents by Guthrie and Johnson (1997) concluded that Graduate Destination Survey figures are likely to be "reasonable indicators of the full-time labour market position of the population of graduates from that relevant cohort."

academic achievement, though this has been examined with similar data by Win and Miller (2005), Birch and Miller (2006a)(2007a)(2007b) and Dobson and Skuja (2005), amongst others. Chia and Miller (2008) did, however, examine starting salaries, though they did not have the detailed focus on age that the current study has. Birch, Li and Miller (2009) also examine graduate starting salaries in Australia, although with different data to that used here.[6] Details on the modelling strategy with respect to both tertiary academic achievement and graduate starting salaries follow.

(A) Model of Tertiary Academic Performance

Students' tertiary academic performance can be modelled within an education production function framework, where academic performance (*Output*) is held to be a function of university enrolment characteristics (*UEC*), and background demographic characteristics (*BC*))[7]. For a given student *i*, the production function can be written as:

$$Output_i = f(UEC_i, BC_i) \quad (1)$$

The measure of tertiary academic performance used in this study is the weighted average mark (WAM) over the entire undergraduate degree program. This differs from the approach taken by Win and Miller (2005), Birch and Miller (2006a)(2007a) and Dobson and Skuja (2005), where the focus is on first-year academic outcomes, and the approach taken by Birch and Miller (2007b), where academic performance over each year of the degree is examined. The more encompassing measure is preferred here simply because it should provide a better assessment of the differences in the academic quality of graduates that employers see at the time of hire. It also provides a more complete coverage of the graduates' academic profiles than does a focus on academic outcomes in particular years of study. The mean WAM is 69.308 (at the border between a Credit and a Distinction), with a standard deviation of 7.180.

There are six university enrolment characteristics (*UEC*) included in the model of tertiary academic performance. The first of these is information on the high school examinations that are used in the university admission decisions for many students (see Appendix A). This information has been shown in past research to be a major determinant of academic outcomes at university. That is, current academic achievements are heavily influenced by earlier academic outcomes, and the most recent information of this type that is available is the best predictor in this regard (Birch and Miller, 2007b). From this perspective, the academic performance in the final year of high school should be a highly relevant predictor of tertiary academic performance in this study. The second enrolment characteristic is the type of attendance at university, namely, whether the graduate attended university on a part-time or full-time basis. Students who attend university on a part-time basis have been associated with

---

6 Birch, Li and Miller (2009) used data on graduates from all Australian universities in 2003 provided by Graduate Careers Australia. They did not have access to information on the students' university records: these data are currently available only if the data are procured from a specific university.

7 Some studies have examined specific environmental factors, such as lecture attendance, characteristics of instructors, study habits and the students' involvement in non-academic activities (*e.g.*, sports, market work). Measures of these are not available in the data set employed here.

poorer academic results in recent research (see, for example, Birch and Miller, 2008). The third enrolment characteristic is the field of study. The influence of field of study has been investigated by a number of studies in Australia (e.g., Everett and Robins, 1991; Cantwell *et al.*, 2001), though the approach adopted and findings reported vary considerably. Nevertheless, it appears from these studies that students enrolled in health and education courses have higher marks at university than students enrolled in maths and science courses.

The final three enrolment characteristics included in the model of tertiary academic performance are intended to capture differences in the type of degree the graduates completed. Thus, these variables record enrolment in an honors degree, a double degree (i.e., where the student completes two degrees simultaneously, such as Arts/Law or Science/Commerce) or a postgraduate bachelor's degree or graduate diploma. The admission criteria for these degrees mean that the students in each of these categories will typically be above average, and hence the variables should each be associated with positive effects in the model of university academic performance.

The background or demographic characteristics included in the model are gender, birthplace and age. Recent studies in Australia have generally reported that female students have better academic results than their male counterparts (e.g., Cantwell *et al.*, 2001). In contrast, the Australian literature has not reached a consensus on the impact that birthplace has on tertiary academic performance (see Birch and Miller (2008) for a review). In this study the birthplace information is combined with information on the year the foreign born arrived in Australia. Thus, immigrants who arrived as young children are distinguished from other immigrants. The age division in this regard (at seven years) is motivated by the research on the critical period hypothesis which suggests there may be a critical (pre-puberty) arrival age where immigrants who arrive before this threshold can develop native-like dominant language fluency.

Mixed findings have been reported on the role that age might have on tertiary academic performance, as has been discussed in Section II. Providing additional information on these age effects is a key focus of the current paper. In this regard, two specifications of the age information are considered. The first is a linear age term. The second is a set of three dummy variables, and this choice is motivated by the research by Klevmarken and Quigley (1976). These age variables differentiate between relatively young students (aged 21 years or under), those who are about average in age (22 to 24 years), and older students (25 years and over).

There are several additional variables included in the models. These cover characteristics of the type of high school attended. In particular, students who attended Independent (i.e., private) or Catholic schools are distinguished from students who attended Government (i.e., State) schools. Furthermore, students who attended small schools are distinguished from students who attended medium and large schools. Finally, a dummy variable is used to capture the influence of attending a co-educational school rather than a single-sex school. Each of these sets of variables, and particularly the first, has been shown to be a significant determinant of academic performance at university in recent research (e.g., Dobson and Skuja, 2005; Birch and Miller, 2007a), with attendance at Independent and Catholic high schools being associated with lower marks at university, and attendance at a co-educational school with higher marks at university.[8]

Thus, the estimating equation used in this study of academic performance at university is specified as:

WAM = f(High School Results, Part-time attendance, Field of study, Honors degree, Double degree, Course type, Gender, Birthplace and Period of arrival, *Age*, Independent, Catholic, Small school, Co-educational school)[9] (2)

(B) Model of Starting Salaries

The model of starting salaries used is a standard earnings equation, with the dependent variable being the log of annual gross salary.

$$\ln(salary)_i = f(X_i) \quad (3)$$

The mean of the dependent variable is 10.214 ($27 282). There is considerable variation in starting salaries, with the standard deviation being 0.908. The explanatory variables (X) included in (3) to account for this variation can be classified into three broad categories, namely personal characteristics, educational profile and employment. The choice of explanatory variables is based on the models of Chia and Miller (2008). Brief descriptions of the main variables follow.

Four personal characteristics are included in the model: gender, birthplace, age at migration and age. The birthplace and age at migration data are combined to form the same foreign born-arrived as children and other foreign born variables that were discussed in relation to the model of university academic performance. In the models estimated on the sample pooled across all age groups, the age information is entered into the model in exponential (Gompertz) form, specifically $e^{-0.1*Age}$. This functional form is generally argued to be superior in the study of young workers, as it avoids the unrealistic prediction of relatively low earnings among groups of middle-aged workers that is associated with the use of a quadratic functional form. In addition, the three dummy variables defined earlier (for students aged 21 years or under, those who are 22 to 24 years, and students 25 years and over) are also used to explore the empirical relevance in Australia of the U-shaped relationship suggested by Klevmarken and Quigley (1976). Most emphasis, however, is placed on the estimation of models on separate samples of younger (defined as less than 25 years of age at graduation) and older (25 or more years of age) graduates.

---

8 There is overlap in the information content of the variables for co-educational schools and Catholic and Independent schools, as only Catholic and Independent schools in the data set are single-sex schools. For this reason results from equations which omit the variable for co-educational school are also discussed.

9 Given the inclusion of variables for high school results and school type, the model also includes dummy variables for cases where this information is not available.

The following descriptors of graduates' education profile are included in the estimating equation: field of study, characteristics of high school, student status at university and academic achievement (i.e., WAM). Variables like these are generally included in studies of graduates' salaries (see Chia and Miller, 2008 for a review). Strong priors, however, cannot be attached to many of the coefficients, though it would be expected that starting salaries will be positively influenced by academic success at university.[10]

There are four variables included in the model to characterise the type of work the graduates do. These are the sector of employment (government, education, private or other, with private sector employees being the omitted category), employment type (permanent or otherwise), study status (dummy for graduates who are studying while working), and occupation (12 broad occupational groups are distinguished). While these variables are likely to be important determinants of graduates' starting salaries, they are not the focus of this study. The results associated with these variables will not, therefore, be reported, but are available upon request from the authors.

Hence, the estimating equation used as the starting point in this research can be written as:

$\ln(salary)$ = f(Gender, Birthplace and Period of arrival, *Age,* WAM, High school results, Part-time attendance, Field of study, Honors degree, Double degree, Course type, Independent, Catholic, Small school, Co-educational school, Characteristics of type of work) (4)

Chia and Miller's (2008) prior analysis of these data revealed that gender, born abroad in an English-speaking country, honors degree, double degree, course type, high school results, co-educational school and a number of variables for the type of work were statistically insignificant.[11] This is also largely a feature of the analysis of much larger samples covering graduates of all universities in Birch, Li and Miller (2009). Accordingly, the restricted specification of Chia and Miller (2008) is followed in this research. This is:

$\ln(salary)$ = f(Birthplace and Period of arrival, *Age*, WAM, Part-time attendance, Field of study, Independent, Catholic, Small school, Characteristics of type of work), (5)

where the birthplace and period of arrival information is restricted to immigrants from non-English-speaking countries.

---

[10] Chia and Miller (2008) show that while there is a strong, positive relationship between graduate starting salaries and academic achievements at university, graduates' high school academic performance is not a statistically significant determinant of starting salaries once university academic performance is accounted for. They argue that this shows that the information content of the high school results is supplanted by the more recent information contained in the data on university academic achievement.

[11] The criterion used in the Chia and Miller (2008) study was a 't' value greater than 1.0. In other words, the inclusion of these statistically insignificant variables would have lowered the adjusted R^2.

IV. EMPIRICAL FINDINGS

(A) Overview of the Data

Table 1 lists the means and standard deviations of the main variables.

Table 1. Descriptive Statistics for Selected Variables, for Total Sample and for those Aged 25 or More Years

Variable	Total Sample	Aged 25+
Weighted Average Mark (WAM)	69.308	69.296
	(7.18)	(7.48)
Log Annual Salary	10.214	10.453
	(0.91)	(0.66)
Linear age (years)	23.545	30.804
	(4.78)	(7.95)
Age < 22 years	0.283	0.000
Age 25+ years	0.171	1.000
Female	0.552	0.559
Born abroad in English-speaking country	0.119	0.172
Born abroad in English-speaking country and arrived as a child	0.059	0.052
Born abroad in non-English-speaking country	0.143	0.131
Born abroad in non-English-speaking country and arrived as a child	0.057	0.035
Honors degree	0.085	0.074
Double degree	0.184	0.063
Postgraduate bachelor's degree or graduate diploma	0.063	0.153
Attended part-time	0.265	0.411
Tertiary Entrance Rank unknown	0.198	0.610
Tertiary Entrance Rank	92.972	93.403
	(5.02)	(3.51)
High school information not available	0.411	0.937
Small high school	0.074	0.022
Independent high school	0.174	0.016
Catholic high school	0.134	0.005
Co-educational high school	0.094	0.003
Sample Size	2143	367

Note: Standard deviations in parentheses for continuous variables only. Information on other variables can be found in Appendix A.

The Table 1 data show that the typical graduate in the sample has completed a standard undergraduate bachelor's degree programme. Three-quarters of the graduates had studied on a full-time basis. For over four-fifths of the sample, there is valid information on the students' tertiary entrance rank (TER). All respondents in the sample have, by construction, information on the WAM at university, and the average of this is almost 70. 8.5 percent of graduates obtained honors, and 18.4 percent of graduates had double degrees. The mean of the natural logarithm of the graduates' starting salaries is 10.214 ($27 282).

Graduates 25 years of age or older differ from other graduates in a number of aspects. They are more likely to pursue qualifications beyond a standard undergraduate bachelor's degree program (15.3 percent had enrolled in a postgraduate bachelor's degree or graduate diploma compared to just 6.3 percent for all graduates). They are more likely to have studied on a part-time basis, with 41 percent of older graduates having part-time student status, compared to 27 percent of all students. This part-time student status itself could account for why these students are older at the time of graduation. Reflecting the different admission categories for many older students, graduates 25 years of age or older are less likely than other graduates to have a TER, with 61 percent of graduates over 25 years old recorded as having an unknown TER, compared to just 20 percent for all graduates.[12] For the same reason, while about three-fifths of the graduates from the full sample had information on their respective high schools, this information was available for less than 10 percent of the graduates over 25 years of age. Only 6 percent of graduates over 25 years old had completed a double degree, lower than the 18 percent for all graduates. These differences in university enrolment characteristics, combined with the age factor itself, presumably go some way to explain why the graduates 25 years of age or older have a relatively high mean annual salary, of 10.453 ($34 648), compared to the mean of 10.214 ($27 282) for all graduates.

(B) Determinants of Tertiary Academic Performance

Results from the estimation of the model of the determinants of tertiary academic performance are presented in Table 2. Column (i) presents results of the analysis on the total sample, and column (iii) presents results from the estimation of the same model of the determinants of tertiary academic performance on the sub-set of graduates who were at least 25 years of age at the time of graduation. The discussion will first focus on the findings in column (i) for all graduates.

Table 2. OLS Estimates of Model of Tertiary Academic Performance[(a)]

Variable	Total Sample (i)	(ii)	25+ years[(c)] (iii)
Constant	13.690	12.322	30.353
	(4.26)	(3.99)	(3.01)
Linear age	-0.047	(b)	(b)
	(1.20)		

[12] Having an unknown TER implies that the graduates had secured admission into the university program by means other than by virtue of a TER. Specifically, they are considered by a selection committee from the respective faculty, which takes into account other qualifications, such as Technical and Further Education or other tertiary results. It is therefore intuitive that this group will be more highly represented in the sample of older graduates. Additional details on the admission process are provided in Appendix A where the Tertiary Entrance Rank variable is described.

Table 2. (Continued)

Variable	Total Sample (i)	(ii)	25+ years[c] (iii)
Age < 22 years	(b)	0.853 (2.51)	(b)
Age 25+ years	(b)	-0.395 (0.82)	(b)
Female	1.602 (5.42)	1.562 (5.29)	1.937 (2.68)
Born abroad in English-speaking country	0.974 (1.74)	0.898 (1.66)	1.426 (1.43)
Born abroad in English-speaking country and arrived as a child	-0.636 (0.83)	-0.539 (0.71)	2.301 (1.32)
Born abroad in non-English-speaking country	-1.383 (2.64)	-1.389 (2.66)	-1.818 (1.28)
Born abroad in non-English-speaking country and arrived as a child	0.305 (0.41)	0.284 (0.38)	-1.321 (0.62)
Architecture	-0.801 (0.99)	-0.726 (0.90)	0.070 (0.04)
Arts	1.766 (1.10)	1.749 (4.07)	2.930 (2.19)
Commerce	-2.004 (4.69)	-2.073 (4.83)	1.181* (0.64)
Computer and Mathematical Science	1.870 (1.56)	1.927 (1.61)	10.268* (4.12)
Economics	-1.680 (1.76)	-1.745 (1.84)	1.592 (0.54)
Dentistry	3.487 (2.43)	3.778 (2.61)	5.890 (1.42)
Engineering	-0.713 (1.33)	-0.567 (1.05)	0.135 (0.08)
Health Science	2.440 (2.89)	2.475 (2.89)	1.229 (0.36)
Law	-4.562 (7.86)	-4.450 (7.63)	-2.536 (1.56)
Medicine	-0.274 (0.51)	-0.025 (0.05)	3.968* (3.11)
Music	2.671 (2.23)	2.746 (2.30)	1.258 (0.72)
Psychology	0.440 (0.38)	0.541 (0.46)	-1.820 (0.87)
Social Work	4.260 (4.91)	4.196 (4.93)	6.969* (5.05)
Honors degree	2.772 (5.45)	2.773 (5.45)	4.334 (3.50)
Double degree	3.347 (7.51)	3.497 (7.61)	5.928 (3.68)

Variable	Total Sample (i)	(ii)	25+ years[c] (iii)
Postgraduate bachelor's degree or graduate diploma	4.850 (7.48)	4.866 (7.58)	4.884 (3.44)
Attended part-time	-2.726 (8.33)	-2.631 (7.98)	-2.218 (2.90)
Tertiary Entrance Rank unknown	0.687 (1.60)	0.708 (1.68)	2.131* (2.80)
Tertiary Entrance Rank	0.608 (17.62)	0.606 (17.56)	0.418* (3.92)
High School Information not available	-0.981 (2.46)	-0.701 (1.66)	-4.013* (2.20)
Small high school	0.333 (0.67)	0.380 (0.76)	-4.722* (1.52)
Independent high school	-1.495 (3.39)	-1.499 (3.41)	-4.555 (1.21)
Catholic high school	-1.069 (2.72)	-1.094 (2.78)	3.109 (0.56)
Co-educational high school	-0.972 (1.89)	-0.937 (1.82)	-1.716 (0.45)
Survey year 2005	0.108 (0.31)	0.217 (0.62)	-1.332* (1.51)
Survey year 2004	0.168 (0.49)	0.236 (0.69)	-1.158* (1.34)
R^2	0.314	0.315	0.249
Sample Size	2143	2143	367

Notes: (a) Absolute value of heteroskedasticity-consistent 't' statistics entered in parentheses; (b) = variable not entered or not relevant; (c) a * against a coefficient indicates that it is significantly different from the coefficients for those aged less than 25 years, with statistical significance being determined from a regression estimated on the entire sample with a full set of interaction terms for the Age 25+ variable.

The adjusted R^2 of 0.314 for column (i) shows that the variables included in this model account for about 31 percent of the variation in the graduates' academic performance around the mean value of 69.308. While the main interest in these results is in the impact of age, a number of the other findings are first discussed in order to establish commonalities with previous studies. This will be useful as the focus in the current set of analyses is on academic performance over the entire degree, whereas the majority of past studies in Australia have had a focus on academic performance in specific years of studies, and particularly the first year of study. Most of the estimates are consistent with findings in the recent studies of university academic performance in Australia (e.g., Dobson and Skuja, (2005), Win and Miller (2005), Birch and Miller (2006a)(2007a) for studies with a focus on first-year university academic outcomes, and Birch and Miller (2005) for separate analyses of academic outcomes in the first, second and third years of university study).

There is a highly significant relationship between tertiary academic performance over the entire degree program and gender, with females having a WAM 1.60 marks higher ('t' = 5.42) than their male counterparts. This marks advantage is at the lower end of the impacts reported in previous studies that have had a focus on single years of study. However, Birch and Miller (2006b) report that the gender differential in academic achievement at university dissipates as later years of study are considered, and so a smaller estimated effect would be expected when the academic performance over the entire degree program, rather than just the first year of study, is considered. This dissipation would be consistent with Tinto's (1975) model of social and economic integration.

The place of birth variables have modest impacts on tertiary academic performance, with graduates born abroad in English-speaking countries (ESB) having average marks about one point greater than the Australian-born reference group (significant at the 10 percent level), and graduates born abroad in non-English-speaking countries (NESB) having a statistically significant academic disadvantage of 1.38 marks. Previous studies in Australia have likewise reported that place of birth has only a minor influence on academic outcomes at university, with the main finding being that students from non-English-speaking countries have outcomes that are slightly inferior to those of other students (see, for example, Birch and Miller, 2008).

The field of study appears to play a part in determining academic results, with over one-half of the field of study variables being statistically significant.[13] The significant effects associated with these variables indicate that there is almost a nine percentage points difference in mean marks across field of study once other university characteristics are held constant. In particular, law is associated with a statistically significant ('t' = 7.86) 4.56 marks disadvantage in academic results, and social work is associated with a 4.26 marks advantage in academic performance ('t' = 4.91). These effects presumably reflect differences in marking practices and expectations across fields of study, together with unmeasured differences between students associated with their choice of particular fields of study.

The type of degree undertaken has a positive impact on academic performance, though this is to be expected given the more stringent admission criteria for some of the degree types. Graduates undertaking an honors degree score 2.77 marks better on average ('t' = 5.45), while double degree holders score 3.35 marks higher ('t' = 7.51) than their peers. Graduates who hold a postgraduate bachelor's or graduate diploma have a 4.85 marks advantage ('t' = 7.48) over graduates with a bachelor's pass degree.

Having studied on a part-time basis is associated with mean marks that are a statistically significant 2.73 percentage points ('t' = 8.33) lower than the reference group of graduates who studied on a full-time basis. As with the findings discussed above, this result for part-time student status is consistent with the literature, where the result is usually interpreted as a consequence of the graduates' other commitments (primarily employment) impacting their study activities. Specialisation in study activities is to be recommended from this perspective.

The TER is shown to have a positive impact on academic performance over the degree program. For every one percentage point increase in the tertiary entrance rank, there is a 0.61 percentage point increase in the WAM. This supports the findings in earlier research, for example, Birch and Miller (2007b), that current academic outcomes are heavily influenced by earlier academic outcomes. Moreover, the fact that the estimated impact in the current set of analyses of academic achievements over the entire degree program is less than the impact of around one reported in Birch and Miller's (2006a)(2007a) studies of academic achievement in

[13] An F-test of the hypothesis that the coefficients on all the field of study variables are simultaneously equal to zero had a value of 13.13, which is highly significant.

the first year reflects the lesser influence the TER has on academic achievements in years of study beyond the first year (see Birch and Miller, 2007b).

High school type plays a part in determining tertiary academic performance as well, with graduates who had attended Independent high schools having mean marks 1.50 points below the mean marks of the benchmark group of graduates who had attended Government schools. Similarly, graduates who had attended Catholic high schools have mean marks that are 1.07 points below those of the benchmark group. Graduates who had attended co-educational high schools have mean marks that are about one point below the mean marks achieved by graduates who had attended single-sex schools. It was noted above that there was overlap in the information content of the type of high schools (i.e., Independent, Catholic) and co-educational high school variables. Hence, the equations were re-estimated omitting the co-educational high school variable. In these equations, the variable for having attended an Independent school was associated with a -1.89 percentage points ('t' = 5.11) effect (compared to the -1.49 effect with the inclusion of the co-education school variable), and the variable for having attended a Catholic school was associated with a -1.24 percentage point ('t' = 3.20) effect (compared to the -1.07 effect in Table 2). Thus, the inclusion of the co-education school variable reduces the impact associated with attending a non-government school, but does not alter the overall assessment of the impact of the type of school on academic outcomes at university.

Turning to the impact of age on academic achievement over the entire degree program, the results in column (i), where age is entered in linear form, suggest that this does not affect how well students perform academically. The estimated coefficient on the linear age variable is small (-0.05) and has a 't' value of only 1.20. In column (ii) of Table 2, however, where two age dummy variables are entered into the model, age is shown to have a significant impact.[14] The difference between the findings in column (i) and those in column (ii) indicate that the effect of age on academic achievements at university is non-linear. The age variable for graduates aged 21 years and below is statistically significant ('t' = 2.5), and shows that these graduates scored, on average, 0.85 marks more than graduates between 22 and 25 years of age. The age variable for graduates above 25 years old is statistically insignificant. Thus, according to these results, students who enter university directly following the completion of high school, and have a normal progression through their program of tertiary studies, have the best academic achievement. However, while their advantage in marks is statistically significant, it is best described as being quite modest.

Column (iii) presents results obtained from the estimation of the model of academic achievement at university on the sub-set of older graduates (i.e., those aged 25 or more years at the time of graduation). The estimates obtained from estimating the model separately for this age group will enable insights into any differences in the determinants of academic success at university that cannot be captured by the intercept shifts that the age dummies represent. The adjusted R^2 for the study of the 25 years plus age group is 0.249, which is lower than when the equation is estimated on a sample pooled across all age groups. The F-test of whether all the coefficients in the model for the 25 years plus age group are

[14] The inclusion of the two age variables in the model increases the adjusted R^2 marginally to 0.315. The signs of the coefficients of the other variables remained unchanged, and additionally, the values of the coefficients remain similar between both models. An F-test of the joint statistical significance of the two age variables has a value of 3.38, which is significant at the three percent level.

simultaneously the same as for the younger ages was a statistically significant 1.97. That is, the hypothesis that the determinants of tertiary academic success for the 25 years and over age group are the same as those that impact the tertiary academic success of the less than 25 years age group can be rejected. Nine of the individual coefficients for the 25 years and over group differ significantly from those estimated for the younger age groups. The variables for the field of study which differ significantly for the older age group are for commerce, computer and mathematical science, medicine, and social work. Graduates who had studied computer and mathematical science are associated with a 10.3 marks advantage, which is about eight marks more than in the analysis for the total sample. In the case of social work, there is a seven percentage point differential in mean marks among the 25 years and older group, which is around three marks more than the marks differential among the full sample.

The effects of the two TER variables (unknown TER and actual TER) also differ significantly for older graduates compared to the respective effects for these two variables among the younger age groups. Older graduates with unknown TER scores do better at university than younger graduates in the same situation (2.13 marks advantage compared to a 0.71 differential in marks). This may mean that the criteria used to admit older students to university (see footnote 12) offer more useful predictors of their academic success. It could also simply mean, however, that the other qualifications used by older students to gain entrance to university are scrutinised more closely, that is, there is a form of institutional selection that is instrumental in generating this finding. The impact of the TER for older graduates is a gain of only 0.42 marks per percentage point increase in the TER, compared with an increase of 0.61 for graduates in the total sample. For older students the TER will generally have been completed some years prior to entering university. Hence, these results reinforce the finding from Birch and Miller (2006b) that the information content of the TER as a predictor of academic outcomes dissipates with the passage of time.

Overall, these analyses show that age, gender, birthplace, degree type, field of study and earlier academic outcomes have substantial effects on tertiary academic performance. Field of study plays a particularly large part in determining academic performance. Age has a limited impact on academic prowess, with younger students, that is, those younger than 22 years of age, faring only marginally better than the 22 to 24 year old group. Importantly, from the perspective of this study, older students (that is, those aged 25 or more years) do just as well, on average, as students 22 to 24 years of age, who make up more than one-half of the student body. Older students can be advantaged by enrolment in computer and mathematical science, medicine and social work, and to a lesser extent in commerce.

(C) Determinants of Starting Salaries

The results of the analysis of the determinants of graduate starting salaries are presented in Table 3. Results from the model used in Chia and Miller (2008) are included in column (i) to provide a reference.[15] This model is based on a Gompertz specification of the age variable (see Appendix A). The model in column (ii) is distinguished by the use of the two age dummies variables described earlier that capture the suggestions of Klevmarken and Quigley

[15] There are minor differences between these results and those in Chia and Miller (2008) owing to the correction of a minor coding error in the earlier study. The changes are not of any material consequence.

(1976) (see Section II(b) above). The different specifications for the age variables across the two models does not lead to any major changes in the fit of the model, or in the estimated coefficients attached to specific variables.

Table 3. OLS Estimates of Model of Graduate Starting Salaries[(a)]

Variable	Total Sample (i)	(ii)	25+ years[(c)] (iii)
Constant	6.953	6.618	6.982
	(34.49)	(36.06)	(18.41)
Age in Gompertz form ($e^{-0.1*age}$)	-3.531	(b)	(b)
	(5.00)		
Age < 22 years	(b)	-0.139	(b)
		(3.64)	
Age 25+ years	(b)	0.137	(b)
		(3.96)	
Born abroad in non-English-speaking	-0.159	-0.156	-0.166
country	(2.48)	(2.42)	(1.71)
Born abroad in non-English-speaking	0.128	0.127	-0.112*
country and arrived as a child	(1.78)	(1.76)	(0.95)
Architecture	0.023	0.015	0.250
	(0.29)	(0.20)	(1.40)
Arts	0.109	0.110	0.168
	(2.08)	(2.09)	(2.00)
Commerce	0.179	0.178	0.297
	(3.38)	(3.32)	(2.80)
Computer and Mathematical Science	0.212	0.202	0.317
	(2.49)	(2.35)	(1.80)
Economics	0.113	0.116	0.396
	(0.53)	(0.54)	(2.42)
Dentistry	0.717	0.669	0.608
	(7.51)	(6.91)	(4.00)
Engineering	0.158	0.152	0.378*
	(2.82)	(2.72)	(2.96)
Health Science	0.240	0.252	0.577*
	(4.12)	(4.26)	(5.94)
Law	0.212	0.201	0.314
	(4.54)	(4.24)	(3.27)
Medicine	0.119	0.088	0.041
	(1.60)	(1.14)	(0.30)
Music	0.308	0.306	-0.330*
	(2.80)	(2.79)	(1.91)
Psychology	0.034	0.023	0.071
	(0.40)	(0.28)	(0.41)
Social Work	0.165	0.214	0.317
	(2.15)	(2.94)	(2.35)

Table 3. (Continued)

Variable	Total Sample (i)	(ii)	25+ years[c] (iii)
Postgraduate bachelor's degree or graduate diploma	0.075	0.091	0.015
	(1.71)	(2.09)	(0.16)
Attended part-time	0.032	0.038	-0.031
	(1.09)	(1.33)	(0.69)
Weighted Average Mark (WAM)	0.007	0.007	0.003
	(4.06)	(4.17)	(1.11)
Tertiary Entrance Rank unknown	-0.115	-0.090	-0.089
	(2.37)	(1.94)	(2.00)
High School Information not available	-0.049	-0.061	0.171
	(1.33)	(1.63)	(1.59)
Small high school	-0.118	-0.123	0.035
	(1.81)	(1.89)	(0.31)
Independent high school	-0.071	-0.070	0.148
	(1.51)	(1.54)	(1.15)
Catholic high school	-0.073	-0.072	0.193
	(1.89)	(1.88)	(1.34)
Survey year 2005	0.096	0.091	0.129
	(3.17)	(2.98)	(2.58)
Survey year 2004	0.016	0.012	-0.004
	(0.54)	(0.41)	(0.08)
Work type variables	Included	Included	Included
R^2	0.629	0.630	0.630
Sample Size	2143	2143	367

Notes: (a) Absolute value of heteroskedasticity-consistent 't' statistics in parentheses; (b) = variable not entered or not relevant; (c) a * against a coefficient indicates that it is significantly different from the coefficients for those aged less than 25 years, with statistical significance being determined from a regression estimated on the entire sample with a full set of interaction terms for the Age 25+ variable.

The adjusted R^2 of the analysis for column (ii) is 0.630, and this shows that this model has considerable explanatory power: Adjusted R^2's of around 0.3 are typical in cross-sectional studies of earnings. In the first instance the variables other than for age are considered, followed by a review of the results for the age variables that are the focus of this set of analysis.

Being born abroad matters to the determination of graduates' starting salaries, but only if the graduates were born in a non-English-speaking country. This group of graduates have earnings around 16 percent[16] less than the earnings of the reference group that comprises of the Australian born and immigrants from English-speaking countries. The coefficient for graduates born abroad in NESB countries, but who arrived in Australia before they turned

[16] For semi-logarithmic regressions, Halvorsen and Palmquist (1980) argue that the interpretation of dummy variables should be calculated by ($e^{\text{coefficient on dummy variable}}$ – 1) x 100. For small values, however, the coefficient itself is a reasonable approximation. For simplicity, the discussion here will be based on the estimated coefficients.

seven years of age, indicates a 13 percent earnings advantage relative to those born abroad in NESB countries who arrived at age seven or older. Thus, this effect more or less offsets the 16 percent birthplace effect, implying that graduates from NESB countries who arrive in Australia as young children have starting salaries comparable to the Australian born.

There is substantial variation, of about 67 percentage points, in graduates' starting salaries across fields of study. Arts graduates earn 11 percent more than the benchmark group of Science graduates, Commerce graduates earn 18 percent more, and Health Science graduates earn 25 percent more than the benchmark group. Dentistry graduates have the highest earnings, with a 67 percent earnings premium relative to the benchmark group of Science graduates. These results are in line with the findings of earlier work, such as Chia and Miller, (2008), and Birch, Li and Miller (2009).

The graduates' WAM results have positive impacts on their starting salaries, with a 0.7 percent increase in earnings for every one mark increase in their WAM (significant at the one percent level). To put this into perspective, a student with a WAM of 50 will earn 25 percent less than a student with a WAM of 85.[17] This equates to roughly three times the size of the reported payoff to a year of schooling in Australia. Clearly there are substantial rewards from having a superior grade point average at university in Australia.

Graduates who had attended a small high school have earnings 12.3 percent below the earnings of graduates who had attended large high schools. There is no obvious reason for this finding, as one would expect any resource or cost-constraints that smaller schools may face to impact high school results rather than labor market outcomes a number of years following graduation from high school. The finding could reflect location issues: to the extent that small schools are disproportionately located in non-metropolitan areas, and these students are subsequently less mobile across regions. However, the same type of finding emerges in the case of the variable for graduates who had attended a Catholic high school, which reveals that these graduates have earnings 7.2 percent lower than graduates who had attended a Government high school.

The estimated coefficients on the two age dummy variables are highly statistically significant. The estimates reveal that graduates less than 22 years of age earn 13.9 percent less than the benchmark group of graduates between 22 and 24 years of age ('t' = 3.64), whereas graduates above 25 years of age earn 13.7 percent more than the benchmark group ('t' = 3.96). Thus, there is a difference in ceteris paribus earnings between the youngest and oldest age groups of almost 28 percent. Additionally, the negative coefficient for graduates younger than 22 years of age (or equivalently, a positive effect for graduates 22 to 24 years compared to graduates under 22 years of age) suggests that the positive effect on earnings of the additional labor market experience of the 22 to 24 year age group dominates any increases in earnings associated with the assumed greater ability of the relatively younger and 'quicker' group. Moreover, omitting the measure of academic achievement (the WAM variable) from the estimating equation changes the estimated age effects by less than one percentage point. This minor change is attributable to the weak links between age and university academic achievement reported in Table 2.

The results from the estimation of the model of graduates' starting salary on a sample restricted to graduates over 25 years of age are reported in column (iii). There are 10 coefficients in the model for these older graduates that differ from the respective coefficients

[17] For a more detailed discussion on the impact of the WAM, see Chia and Miller (2008).

for graduates under 25 years of age. However, these differences are typically minor, and five of them are significantly different from zero only at the 10 percent level of significance. An F-test of whether all differences between the estimated coefficients for those over 25 years of age and those under 25 years of age are simultaneously equal to zero—that is, whether the models for the determinants of starting salaries among these two age groups are the same—had a test statistic of just 1.22, which is insignificant. In other words, the model for the determinants of starting salaries among those 25 years of age or older is the same as that which is applicable to graduates under 25 years of age. Consequently, only brief comments on specific differences in coefficients are provided.

Being born abroad in a NESB country, and arriving in Australia as a child, is associated with a 12.7 percent advantage in the full sample analysis. However, when the sample was restricted to graduates over 25 years old, this earnings premium became an earnings deficit of 11.2 percent. Engineering graduates had an earnings premium of 37.8 percent among the group of older graduates, an advantage more than double the 15.2 percent premium in the full sample analysis. Likewise, the earnings advantage for health science graduates doubled from 25.2 percent to 57.7 percent. Music graduates, on the other hand, who were associated with an earnings advantage of 30.6 percent in the full sample, were associated with an earnings disadvantage of 33 percent compared to the benchmark group of science graduates.

In summary, these analyses show that age is a strong determinant of graduates starting salaries, accounting for an earnings variation of almost 28 percent. The positive relationship between age and starting salaries suggests that labor market experience is relatively important in determining earnings, compared to ability, at least in the beginning of the individual graduate's career.

V. Summary and Conclusion

The analyses of academic achievement at university reported in this paper show that students whose age at graduation indicated that they have entered university directly from high school and have experienced a normal progression through their bachelor's degree program (28 percent of the sample) have superior academic performance to other students. However, their advantage in this regard is less than one percentage point. Mature-age students (17 percent of the sample) have academic achievements over the course of their degree program that cannot be distinguished statistically from the academic outcomes of the majority of students aged 22-24 years of age at graduation. There is some evidence, however, that mature-age students can do better by enrolling in computer and mathematical science, medicine, social work, and to a lesser extent, commerce, courses.

Graduates aged 25 or more years at the time of graduation have earnings about 14 percent more than graduates aged 22 to 24 years at graduation. In turn, graduates aged 22 to 24 years at graduation have earnings about 14 percent more than their counterparts who were under 22 years of age when they graduated. This effect is likely to reflect the impact on earnings of labor market experience. Thus, mature-age students (i.e. those aged 25 or more years at graduation) have earnings about 28 percent higher than the typical direct entry student when other factors, including academic achievements at university, are held constant. The starting salaries of mature-age students appear to be determined in the same way as the starting salaries of other students.

Thus, these results suggest that mature-age students can compete successfully with younger students at university. They outperform younger students in the labor market. If the future progress of a nation depends on providing opportunities for older adults to upgrade and refresh their skills (see Section I), these analyses suggest that the university sector in Australia is doing this very effectively at present. This would auger well for expansion of opportunities for older adults in the tertiary sector. Expansion of mature-age enrolments in the fields of computer and mathematical science, medicine, social work, and commerce may be particularly beneficial.

APPENDIX A
DEFINITION OF VARIABLES

The data are from two sources: the Student Records System at the University of Western Australia, and the Graduate Destination Survey of graduates from this University. Details on the variables formed are presented below.

Age: This is the graduate's age on 30 April in the survey year. The mean age was 23.5 years. The age information is used in three ways. First, a linear age variable is used in some of the estimating equations in the study of the determinants of academic achievements at university. Second, the age variable is used in Gompertz form ($e^{-0.1*Age}$) in some of the estimating equations in the study of the determinants of graduates' starting salaries. Third, age dummies for less than 22 years of age (28.3 percent of the sample), 22-24 years of age (54.6 percent of the sample) and age 25 or more years (17.1 percent of the sample) are used in both sets of analyses.

Country of Birth: The detail on country of birth is aggregated to form three broad birthplace categories: the Australian born; immigrants from the main English-speaking countries; and immigrants from other (non-English-speaking) countries, and dichotomous variables are used for the latter two groups. 11.9 percent of the sample was born abroad in English-speaking countries and 14.3 percent of the sample was born abroad in non-English-speaking countries. The Australian born are used as the reference group in the study of academic performance at university, and the Australian born and immigrants from the main English-speaking countries are used as the reference group in the analysis of graduates' starting salaries.

Age at Migration: Reflecting some of the recent literature on the critical period hypothesis (see, for example, Chiswick and Miller, 2008), a dummy variable was formed for immigrants who arrived in Australia before they were seven years of age. The argument underlying this variable is that immigrants who arrive as young children but not those who arrive at an older age can be expected to develop "Native-like" proficiency in English. This variable has a mean of 0.059 for immigrants from English-speaking countries, and a mean of 0.057 for immigrants from non-English-speaking countries.

Female: The gender dichotomous variable is defined to equal one for females and to equal zero for males. 55.2 percent of the sample are females.

Weighted Average Mark (WAM): This is the average of the marks in each unit of study towards the degree, weighted by the relative importance of each unit in the degree program. For example, if the student enrolled in 24 "six-point" units as part of their degree, then each would be given equal weight. If, however, they enrolled in 20 "six-point" units and two "12-point" units, the latter two units would be given twice the weight of the first 20. The mean WAM is 69.308. It has a standard deviation of 7.180.

Honors Degree: This is a dummy variable, defined to equal one for students who completed an honors degree (8.5 percent of the sample), and defined to equal zero for students who completed a pass degree. An honors degree is usually an additional year of study following the completion of a pass degree, though for some fields of study it is awarded to reflect a standard of achievement over the degree program.

Double Degree: This is a dummy variable, defined to equal one for students who completed a double degree (that is, studied for two degrees simultaneously, such as Law/Commerce, Law/Arts) and defined to equal zero for students who completed a single degree. 18.4 percent of the sample completed double degrees.

Course Type: The focus of the study is on bachelor's degree students. While this is a reasonably homogeneous group, there are some differences that need to be accommodated in the statistical analyses. Hence graduates who completed a postgraduate bachelor's or graduate diploma (6.3 percent of the sample) are distinguished through a dummy variable from students who have completed only a standard undergraduate degree.

Attendance Type: Graduates who studied on a part-time basis (26.5 percent of the sample) are distinguished from those who studied on a full-time basis.

Tertiary Entrance Rank (TER): Students gain entry into the University of Western Australia in two ways. First, if they complete high school in the five years prior to admission, their results in the Tertiary Entrance Examination (the final examination in high school, which has a 50 percent external examination component and a 50 percent school assessment component) in Western Australia, or the equivalent interstate or New Zealand examination, are used in the entrance decision. Second, all other applicants are considered by the relevant faculty selection committee on an individual basis. While these could be admitted based on the standard high school examinations, many are admitted on the basis of other qualifications. They will not have a TER and are assigned a value of one on the "unknown TER" dummy variable. 19.8 percent of the sample are in this category. The TER is the student's rank in the high school cohort, such that a value like 99.50 indicates that the student's results are better than the results of 99.50 percent of the cohort. The maximum value of the variable is 99.95.

High School Unknown: Information on the type of school attended is included in the model where it is available. For 41.1 percent of the sample, however, this information is not available. A dichotomous variable is used to represent these graduates in the estimating equation.

High School Size: Students who attended a high school that had 100 or fewer students in their final year of study (7.4 percent of the graduates) are distinguished from other graduates through a dummy variable. Students who attended medium and large high schools are the reference group.

High School Type: There are three broad types of high schools: Independent, Catholic and Government. Dichotomous variables for the first two categories of schools (with means of 17.4 percent and 13.4 percent, respectively) are used to capture this information. Students who attended Government schools are the reference group.

Co-educational School: A dummy variable is used to distinguish students who had attended a co-educational high school (9.4 percent of the sample) from students who had attended a single-sex high school.

Field of Study: Dummy variables are used in the analysis for the major fields of study. These are (with means in parentheses): Architecture (4.1 percent), Arts (13.1 percent), Commerce (14.7 percent), Computer and mathematical science (2.3 percent), Dentistry (1.9 percent), Economics (2.3 percent), Engineering (17.0 percent), Health sciences (1.2 percent), Law (7.8 percent), Medicine (7.0 percent), Music (1.7 percent), Psychology (0.8 percent) and Social work (2.2 percent). The omitted category is the 23.9 percent of graduates who completed a degree in Science.

Year of Graduation: As the survey contains data from 2003, 2004 and 2005, dummy variables are used to identify graduates who were surveyed in 2005 (41.5 percent) and 2004 (29.2 percent). Graduates who were surveyed in 2003 (29.3 percent) are the reference group.

Starting Salary: This is the natural logarithm of annual gross wage/salary, as reported in the Graduate Destination Survey. It has a mean of 10.214 ($27 282). The standard deviation of the starting salary variable is 0.908.

Sector of Employment: Four broad employment sectors were formed: Government (23.3 percent of graduates), Education (9.2 percent of graduates), Private (58.8 percent) and Other, which includes the self-employed and those employed in the not-for-profit sector (8.6 percent). Private sector employees are the reference group.

Employment Type: Information is available on whether employed graduates were permanent or anticipated being with their employer for 12 months or more. These graduates (67.7 percent) are distinguished from other graduates using a dummy variable.

Study Status: A dummy variable is used for graduates who were still studying at the time of the survey (27.9 percent). The omitted category is graduates who were not studying anymore.

Occupation: Dummy variables are included in the earnings equation for employment as: Managers or administrators (2.1 percent), Natural and physical science professionals (7.3 percent), Building and engineering professionals (16.0 percent), Accounting professionals (6.5 percent), Business and information professionals (8.7 percent), Health professionals (9.8 percent), Education professionals (6.8 percent), Social, arts and miscellaneous professionals (6.0 percent), Associate professionals (9.4 percent), Other occupations (2.3 percent), Advanced clerical and service workers (3.1 percent) and Intermediate or elementary clerical, sales and service workers (21.7 percent). The final occupation listed here is used as the reference group in the statistical analyses.

REFERENCES

Bedard, K and Dhuey, E., (2006). "The Persistence of Early Childhood Maturity: International Evidence of Long-Run Age Effects", *The Quarterly Journal of Economics*, pp.1437-1472.

Birch, E. R., Li, I. and Miller, P. W., (2009). "The Influences of Institution Attended and Field of Study on Graduates' Starting Salaries", *Australian Economic Review*, Vol. 42, No. 1, pp.42-63.

Birch, E. R. and Miller, P. W., (2006a). "Student Outcomes at University in Australia: A Quantile Regression Approach", *Australian Economic Papers*, Vol. 45, No. 1, pp.1-17.

Birch, E. R. and Miller, P. W., (2006b). "The Impact of HECS Debt on Australian Students' Tertiary Academic Performance", *Education Research and Perspectives*, Vol. 33, No. 1, pp.1-32.

Birch, E. R. and Miller, P. W., (2007a). "The Influence of Type of High School Attended on University Performance", *Australian Economic Papers*, Vol. 46, No. 1, pp.1-17.

Birch, E. R. and Miller, P. W., (2007b). "Tertiary Entrance Scores: Can We Do Better?", *Education Research and Perspectives*, Vol. 34, No. 2, pp.1-23.

Birch, E. R. and Miller, P. W., (2008). "A National Study of Student Outcomes at University", *Australasian Journal of Economics Education*, (forthcoming).

Byrd, R., Weitzmanm, M. and Auinger, P., (1997). "Increased Behavior Problems Associated with Delayed School Entry and Delayed School Progress", *Pediatrics*, Vol. 100, pp.654-661.

Cantwell, R., Archer, J. and Bourke, S., (2001). "A Comparison of the Academic Experiences and Achievement of University Students Entering by Traditional and Non-Traditional Means", *Assessment and Evaluation in Higher Education*, Vol. 26, No. 3, pp. 221-234.

Chia, G. and Miller, P. W., (2008). "Tertiary Performance, Field of Study, and Graduate Starting Salaries", *Australian Economic Review*, Vol. 41, No. 1, pp.15-31.

Chiswick, B. R. and Miller, P. W., (2008). "A Test of the Critical Period Hypothesis for Language Learning", *Journal of Multilingual and Multicultural Development*, Vol. 29, No. 1, pp.16-29.

Datar, A., (2006). "Does Delaying Kindergarten Entrance Give Children a Head Start?", *Economics of Education Review*, Vol. 25, pp.43-62.

Del Bono, E. and Galindo-Rueda, F., (2004). "Do a Few Months of Compulsory Schooling Matter? The Education and Labour Market Impact of School Leaving Rules", Institute for the Study of Labor, Bonn, Discussion Paper No. 1233.

Department of Education, Employment and Workplace Relations, (2008). Review of Australian Higher Education, Discussion Paper, Department of Education, Employment and Workplace Relations, Canberra, June.

Department of Education, Employment and Workplace Relations, (2009). *Publications and Resources Main Page*, Available from: http://www.dest.gov.au/common_topics /publications_resources/default.htm [21st January 2009].

Dickson, J., Fleet, A. and Watt, H., (2000). "Success or Failure in a Core University Unit: What Makes a Difference", *Higher Education Research and Development*, Vol. 19, No. 1, pp.59-73.

Dobson, I. and Skuja, E., (2005). "Secondary Schooling, Tertiary Entrance Ranks and University Performance", *People and Place*, Vol. 13, No. 1, pp.53-62.

Duncan, O. D., (1961). "A Socioeconomic Index for All Occupations", in Albert J. Reiss Jr (ed.), *Occupational and Social Status*, New York: Free Press, pp.109-138.

Everett, J. and Robins, J., (1991). "Tertiary Entrance Predictors of First-year University Performance", *Australian Journal of Education*, Vol. 35, No. 1, pp.24-40.

Fredriksson, P. and Ockert, B., (2005). "Is Early Learning Really More Productive? The Effect of School Starting Age on School and Labour Market Performance", Institute for the Study of Labor, Bonn, Discussion Paper No. 1659.

Goodman, A. and Sianesi, B., (2005). "Early Education and Children's Outcomes: How Long do the Impacts Last?", *Fiscal Studies*, Vol. 26, pp.513-548.

Graduate Careers Australia., (2009). *GradStats and GradFiles, gradlink: graduate careers and employment,* [Online], Graduate Careers Australia. Available from: *http://www.graduatecareers.com.au/content/view/full/24* [15 March 2006].

Graue, E. and DiPerna, J., (2000). "Redshirting and Early Retention: Who gets the 'Gift of Time' and What are its Outcomes?", *American Education Review Journal*, Vol. 37, pp.507-534.

Guthrie, B. and Johnson, T., (1997). *Study of Non-Response to the 1996 Graduate Destination Survey,* [Online], Department of Employment, Education, Training and Youth Affairs. Available from: http://www.dest.gov.au/archive/highered /eippubs /eip9710/front.htm#contents [2 April 2006].

Halvorsen, R. and Palmquist, R., (1980). "The Interpretation of Dummy Variables in Semilogarithmic Equations", *American Economic Review*, Vol. 70, No. 3, pp. 474-475.

Klevmarken, A. and Quigley, J. M., (1976). "Age, Experience, Earnings, and Investments in Human Capital", *Journal of Political Economy*, Vol. 84, No. 1, pp.47-72.

Langer, P., Kalk, J. and Searls, D., (1984). "Age of Admission and Trends in Achievement: A Comparison of Blacks and Caucasians", *American Educational Research Journal*, Vol. 21, pp.61-78.

Le, A. T., Miller, P. W., Heath, A. and Martin, N., (2005). "Early Childhood Behaviours, Schooling and Labour Market Outcomes: Estimates from a Sample of Twins", *Economics of Education Review*, Vol. 24, No. 1, pp.1-17.

Long, M., Faust, B., Harris, J., King, B., Knight, A. and Taylor, J., (1994). "A Study of the Academic Results of On-Campus and Off-Campus Students: Comparative Performance Within Four Australian Tertiary Institutions', National Board of Employment, Education and Training Commissioned Report No. 34, Australian Council for Education, Employment and Training, Canberra, Australia.

McKenzie, K. and Schweitzer, R., (2001). "Who Succeeds at University? Factors Predicting Academic Performance in First Year Australian University Students", *Higher Educational Research and Development*, Vol. 20, No. 1, pp.21-33.

May, D., Kundert, D. and Brent, D., (1995). "Does Delayed School Entry Reduce Later Grade Retentions and Use of Special Education Services?", *Remedial and Special Education*, Vol. 16, pp.288-294.

Smyth, G., Knuiman, M., Thornett, M. and Kilveri, H., (1990). "Using the EM Algorithm to Predict First-Year University Performance", *Australian Journal of Education*, Vol. 34, No. 2, pp.204-234.

Stipek, D. and Byler, P., (2001). "Academic Achievement and Social Behaviours Associated With Age of Entry into Kindergarten", *Applied Developmental Psychology*, Vol. 22, pp.175-189.

Tinto, V., (1975). "Dropout from Higher Education: A Theoretical Synthesis of Recent Research", *Review of Educational Research*, Vol. 45, No. 1, pp.89-125.

Win, R. and Miller, P. W., (2005). "The Effects of Individual and School Factors on University Students' Academic Performance", *Australian Economic Review*, Vol. 38, No.1, pp.1-18.

In: New Research in Education Adult, Medical and Vocational ISBN 978-1-60741-873-3
Editors: Edmondo Balistrieri and Giustino DeNino © 2009 Nova Science Publishers, Inc.

Chapter 2

TRANSFORMING CHINA'S ADULT AND CONTINUING EDUCATION: STRUCTURE, MANAGEMENT, AND QUALITY

Ning Rong Liu
College of Humanities and Law, School of Professional and Continuing Education, The University of Hong Kong[1], Hong Kong, China

ABSTRACT

China's adult and continuing education has undergone dramatic changes in recent years following the rapid expansion of enrollment in universities. This article examines strategies and approaches that adult and continuing education in China has responded to the challenges and opportunities. It first attempts to provide a critical review of neoliberal policies of marketization in higher education. Then historical perspectives of adult and continuing education in China are given, and this analysis is aimed at contributing to a better understanding of the development of China's adult and continuing education sector. Following this review, the strategies of responses are explored in detail to examine how the restructuring has impacted on the adult higher education system and institutional structure, which in turn will decide whether educators in adult and continuing education can efficiently address the relevant needs in this changing economic and social environment and provide the high quality of professional continuing education programs. It concludes that the strategies adopted by adult and continuing education in China have been consistent with the global trend of marketization in higher education.

Keywords: adult and continuing education, structure, management, quality, China

---

[1] Room 1009, T T Tsui Building, The University of Hong Kong, Pokfulam Rd., Hong Kong, China Email: nr.liu@hkuspace.hku.hk.

INTRODUCTION

There were two parallel higher education systems existing side-by-side in China—regular higher education and adult higher education. While regular institutions of higher education admit secondary school graduates who pass the national college entrance examination, adult institutions of higher education enroll working adults to meet the huge demand for postsecondary studies. An important consideration in establishing adult institutions of higher education was to provide additional opportunities for adults to attain higher education since the resources available in the universities were scarce and thus could only admit a limited number of secondary school graduates. In this sense, adult higher education in China generally refers to any studies leading to a first degree of diploma provided to working adults. This proved to be effective in developing countries as a way to supplement the regular higher education system and to provide working adults with higher education opportunities.

This dual system of higher education functioned well in the 1980s and 1990s. However, the picture shifted towards the end of the last century when the Chinese government promoted the massification of higher education. In response to the demand for higher education, in 1998 the Chinese government decided to increase the enrollment numbers for the universities. As a result of the policy change, higher education expanded at an unprecedented speed. In 2005, the total number of new students increased from 1.08 million in 1994 to 5.3 million in 2006, creating one of the largest higher education systems in the world.

With the dramatically rising enrollment of new students in regular institutions of higher education, adult institutions of higher education feared that they would lose their competitive edge and face decreasing enrollments. Adult higher education in China has long been recognized as a means for upgrading the work force and has also been advocated as an alternative for promoting the expansion of higher education. However, the quality of many programmes in general may not maintain the same high standards. The transformation of traditional adult higher education institutions thus gained a new momentum in the new millennium and adult higher education must be steered to a new direction for the further development. After more than two decades of socialist-market reforms in China, the public and private demand for human capital has also increased rapidly. A range of new education-related opportunities have therefore sprung up for adult institutions of higher education to provide market-oriented programs to train executives and professionals. This has become a major engine for the growth of the adult higher education sector. Adult institutions of higher education have expanded the scope of operation and changed the primary focus from offering degree programs to professional continuing education programs. Thus, the restructuring of adult institutions of higher education in China has created a new emphasis on continuing professional education instead of providing academic degree programmes for working adults.

The new orientation has much broader implications that clearly shift the function and purposes of adult higher education. This emphasizes the assumption that adult education institutions must respond to market needs quickly and create more learning opportunities to upgrade the skills and knowledge of working professionals. In this context, adult higher education institutions are called upon to do more to meet the demands of social and economic development, and, to do this, it is argued that its operations need to be more market-oriented.

HIGHER EDUCATION AND THE MARKET

During the last two decades of the twentieth century, markets came progressively to be seen as the most desirable mechanism for regulating economies and reforming the public sector. The right-wing ascendancy began in the late 1970s in the US with the Reagan neoliberal program of small government, tax cuts, deregulation, and free trade. The neoliberal agenda in the UK started to dominate in a powerful platform after Margaret Thatcher came to power. This trend continued to spread after national governments of both left and right implemented a wave of reforms—privatizations, dismantling of social welfare apparatuses, retreat of the state from economic regulation, tax cuts, deregulation, opening of national boundaries—that profoundly transformed the relationship between their citizens, the state and the economy (Campbell and Peterson, 2001).

The movement of public services into direct competition with their private enterprise counterparts is a common feature of public sector policy throughout the developed world. The publicly funded provision of education has not been exempt from this trend. The ascendancy of neoliberalism and the associated discourse of the new public management, during the 1980s and 1990s have produced a fundamental shift in the way universities have defined and justified their institutional existence (Olssen and Peters, 2005). Neoliberal policies of marketization in education are rooted in postmodernism. The "rapid rise of the market form in education is best understood as a post-modern phenomenon" (Kenway, 1992, p.12), and "the logic of the postmodern argument points towards an individualistic educational consumerism in many respects similar to that advocated by the free-marketers of the new Right" (Green, 1997, p.20).

The term "neoliberalism" is also called "economic rationalism", and it has dominated the way public policy is made and managed in many developed countries. "Economic rationalism" assumes that "the market will deliver the best outcomes because consumers can be counted on to act rationally in making their choices and purchases" (Baldwin and James, 2000, p.140). Neoliberals claim that the invisible hand of the market will inexorably lead to better outcomes in education. "Underlying neoliberal policies in education and their social policies in general is a faith in the essential fairness and justice of markets' (Apple, 1999, p. 207). For neoliberals, consumer choice is crucial and students can make a choice among a vast array of education products. Based on neoliberal economics, it is argued that education should not be paid for through taxation, and that educational institutions should be deregulated in order to compete fairly in the market for the dollar of students/clients.

The reform agenda in education, therefore, is oriented to the market rather than to public ownership or to governmental planning and regulation. In order to improve their competitiveness and effectiveness, schools and universities are seen to need to restructure themselves and adopt marketization as their governance strategies. This trend is especially manifest in higher education (Tiffin and Rajasingham, 1995). The impact of marketization on higher education has driven faculty to become entrepreneurs (Slaughter and Leslie, 1997), and universities have increasingly adopted market-oriented principles and business-like criteria (Currie, 1998). Further, as Clark (1998) concludes, many universities, by means of entrepreneurial action, have transformed themselves.

While the government is still often a big player in higher education, market forces have dramatically increased the institutional influence. One visible change in such education reforms is the decline of professional dominance and the rise of consumerism—the belief that consumers have a right to express their views about services and that their knowledge and opinions have value and validity (Bridges, 1994). As Kwiek clearly points out, "higher education is asked to adapt to new societal needs, to be more responsive to the world around it, to be more market-, performance-, and student-oriented, to be more cost-effective, accountable to its stakeholders, as well as competitive with other providers" (Kwiek, 2003, p. 82).

However, there is no clear evidence to confirm the claims that marketization can lead to a higher achieving educational system (Green, 1997). Even long before the global trend of marketization of education, Blaug raised a number of significant questions about the potential risk, stating that "we have too little experience with the market provision of education to predict the precise effect of enhanced choice backed up by purchasing power, and to argue that competition will necessarily improve education as it has improved the quality of automobiles is mere dogma" (Blaug, 1970, p. 314). By contrast, there is increasing empirical evidence that the development of 'quasi-markets' in education has led to the exacerbation of existing class and racial social divisions (Whitty, Power, and Halpin, 1998; Lauder and Hughes, 1999). Thus, neoliberal policies can create inequality in education (Apple, 2001).

Adult Higher Education in China: Historical Perspectives

Many scholars have emphasized the significant linkages between education and politics. It is widely recognized that the state has a major role in shaping policies and practices in education (Evans, Rusechemeyer, Skocpol, 1985), and the political character of the state determines the nature of the education it offers (Kandel, 1933). "Politics and education live in a symbiotic relationship, with each influencing the fate of the other" (Thomas, 1983, p. 1). This is even more evident in China, where educational policies have a profound impact on the development of adult education ranging from its structure and management, to teaching and learning.

For almost a half-century, since the founding of the People's Republic of China in 1949, the Chinese government adopted the strategy of expanding regular higher education and simultaneously developing adult higher education. By doing so, China attempted to address the dilemma relating to the enormous demand for talent and the underdeveloped higher education system. The large scale of adult higher education had implications in two main areas. While it contributed towards the expansion of higher education, it also played an important role in China's economic development by providing necessary and qualified manpower.

Adult Higher Education and Manpower Training

The Chinese government is explicit about the link between education and economic development, and related education to serve the nation's modernization (Hayhoe, 1992). It has long viewed adult education as critical to the economic development and modernization process. Adult higher education played a very important role in training employed personal, enhancing the quality of current workers, and scientists, government officials and industrial leaders. Thus, China's education policy makers and educators in recent years adopted the concept of lifelong learning to primarily address the needs of economic growth and increased productivity, with less importance attached to create conditions of social progress. By accepting human capital perspectives of lifelong learning, China's education policy makers hoped to form a long-term policy, which in turn could provide the well-trained talents in order to compete in the global economy.

The development of adult higher education in China could be divided into three phases—the pre-reform period (1949-1978), the formalization of adult higher education (1979-1992), and the era of lifelong learning (1993-Present). Its progress always interweaved with the political events and economic development of the time.

1. The Pre-Reform Period (1949-1978)

Immediately after the founding of People's Republic of China in 1949, the Chinese leaders at the time declared that socialist construction would be the main task of this newly established state. They wasted no time to propose and implement a series of education reforms in order to lead China out of poor and backward conditions. The First Conference on Higher Education was held in June 1950, and it stressed that higher education must keep close pace with the needs of national construction. This principle also guided the development of adult higher education.

An extensive restructuring of the existing higher education institutions began in 1950, and it was regarded equally important to put efforts into developing adult higher education. Universities and colleges set up the correspondence programs and evening schools in order to accommodate the demand for higher education among working adults in the 1950s. On the eve of the Cultural Revolution which started in 1966, the correspondence programs claimed to attract 190,000 students and the evening schools enrolled almost 18,000 students. These figures counted as being one-forth of the total enrollment numbers of regular higher education institutions at the time (China Education Yearbook 1949-1981, 1984). However, the development of adult higher education came to a halt, when the Cultural Revolution erupted and plunged China into turmoil for ten years from 1966 to 1976.

2. Formalization of Adult Higher Education (1979-1992)

When China launched economic reforms and decided to open the door to foreign investment after the third Plenary of the Eleventh Congress of the Chinese Communist Party (CCP) in December 1978, the country lacked the skilled and professional people needed for its modernization in the new era. Between the mid-1960s and 1976, the proportion of technicians in the industrial labor force declined from 4% to 2.6% (Naughton, 1995). The national college entrance examination was resumed after ten-years of radical ideology, and the first group of students started their undergraduate studies in the Spring of 1978. Despite the efforts made and the leap in enrollment in universities and colleges, China experienced a great shortfall of places for postsecondary education in the 1980s owing to the increasing demand for higher education.

Seeing the future potential, the government launched reforms for adult higher education. The First National Conference of Adult Education was held in 1986 to discuss the role of adult education in economic development. In the following year, the government released the first policy initiative on adult education, and the document entitled "Decision on Development and Reform of Adult Education" pronounced that advancement of education levels of the whole society were critical to the cause of social modernization (State Council, 1987). The Chinese government attempted to develop adult higher education in the service of modernization. Most universities and colleges also set up schools of adult education to coordinate all higher education programs for adult students and to assure the quality of the programs. China's adult education entered into a new era of rapid growth.

3. The Era of Lifelong Learning (1993-Present)

The year 1993 witnessed the beginning of the comprehensive refurbishment of China's adult higher education. The Outline for Reform and Development of Education in China issued by CCP and the State Council on February 13, stated clearly that adult education is a newly developed system which would lead to lifelong education from traditional education, and it called for building a lifelong learning system with its focus on providing continuing education and on-job training programs (CCPCC and State Council, 1993). As a result, the committee of continuing education in higher education institutions was formed by the central government. In anticipation of the changes in the new millennium, the Ministry of Education in December 1998 proposed an 'Action Plan to Revitalize Education Towards the Twenty-First Century' to establish a lifelong learning system by 2010 (MoE, 1998). The term lifelong learning as opposed to adult education began to infiltrate Chinese policy documents, and the government adopted the framework of lifelong learning, reflecting the international trend.

The development of higher education in the late 1990s marked a dramatic policy change shifting from elite higher education to mass higher education. In 1998, the Chinese government decided to increase the ratio of gross enrollment from 9% to 15% by 2010 (CCPCC and State Council, 1998). However the goal was accomplished by 2003. As a result, in 1999 the MoE called upon adult institutions of higher education to shift their focus from offering degree-oriented programs to launching continuing professional education programs. With the emphasis on continuing education, universities in China started to rename their schools of adult education to schools of continuing education.

The Pioneer of Higher Education Reforms

The Chinese higher education system has reacted to globalization and the knowledge economy in ways common to other counties (Postiglione, 2003). Facing the challenge of global economic integration and the knowledge economy, the Chinese government has adopted the two strategies of decentralization and marketization in restructuring higher education. These dual approaches have imposed a great impact on the governance of higher education in China (Yin and White, 1994). Higher education is increasingly seen as a channel for social mobility and personal development, and the government has begun to see higher education as consumption and a private good benefiting primarily the individual (Ngok and Kwong, 2003).

Prior to the 1985 reform of the education system, China's higher education was highly centralized, and coincided with the Soviet style planned economy. The organizational structure of China's higher education was to make sure that the Communist Party could assume all-encompassing control. The government decided and controlled almost every aspect of higher education—admission criteria and enrollment number, curriculum and teaching material, subject offered and new program approval, staff appointment and financial allocation, tuition fees and job assignment upon graduation, and others.

Education reform in China gained momentum in 1993, which started a new era of higher education reform. A series of reforms were launched changing the funding allocation system for universities and requiring the local governments to provide financial support to universities in their jurisdictions (Agelasto and Adamson, 1998; Wang, 2001; Mok, 2002). A free higher education system was altered by conducting experiments for charging students tuition fees in some universities. The reform underscored the importance of changing the government function from the direct control of managing universities by focusing on policy-making and long-term planning and expanding autonomy for universities. The decentralization of higher education went further in broader areas with the support from the central government.

The adoption of decentralization thus increased the degree of autonomy and flexibility for universities in governance and management. An investigation in late 1998 revealed that universities in China gained more autonomous rights in the following areas: universities had more room to develop courses based on the needs of the market and their own internal considerations, to set up organizational structures when necessary, and to make appointments of or dismiss university staff (Bie, 1999). However, there were some concerns that needed to be addressed and there existed areas that required further improvement—universities did not have enough autonomous rights in deciding admission criteria and enrollments, setting up specialized subjects, designing course content, and granting student diplomas (Li, 2000).

In this context of higher education reform, adult higher education in China was sometimes seen as an experimental field used to restructure the higher education sector. It can be said that adult higher education started the process of marketization and decentralization of higher education in China.

Firstly, the development of adult higher education was the result of a timely response to the market needs for higher education, which arose right after the era of the open-door policy. It could be divided into two different periods in term of its target students. Adult higher education mainly functioned to help those who lost educational opportunities during the Culture Revolution when the majority of students were working adults before the mid-1980s. While the needs of this group of students were met, educators immediately turned to those secondary school graduates who could not get into the regular higher education institutions due to the very limited number of enrollments set by the central government. Adult higher education offered them a second chance to pursue higher education. In other words, the development and rapid growth of adult higher education took advantage of the incapability of the higher education sector to meet market demands, and it challenged the constraints of highly centralized structures in regular higher education institutions.

Secondly, the reform of higher education financing originated in adult higher education. While higher education was seen as the government's responsibility to its citizens in the late 1970s, students who participated in adult higher education programs either paid on their own or their working units reimbursed them for their studies. In 1985, two types of students were allowed to be enrolled in adult higher education programs. One was contract students who were selected by the company to study in colleges, and another was self-financed students. Not until 1993 were 30 higher education institutions given the authority to carry out experiments with fee-paying schemes which allowed students to enroll in universities with lower scores by paying tuition fees. By 1997, all students in higher education institutions would need to pay tuition fees. This departed from almost five decades of free higher education in China. It was the adult higher education system which first generated such funds for universities, because they were not allocated finances by the central government.

Thirdly, adult higher education started to develop in full-scale when universities and colleges were still closed to the society. Since higher education developments prior to the reform era were decided and planned by the central government, universities were left no room to operate according to political, economic, and social developments. The development of adult higher education thus helped change the structures of higher education institutions in China, which in general did not emphasize the importance of linking what they taught in classrooms with needs in society. Since the majority of adult learners had some working experience, adult and continuing education was subject to external influences on its development. All in all, adult higher education helped Chinese universities to build much closer links with the economy and the society.

Poor Quality of Adult Higher Education Programs

While adult higher education gave much priority to degree programs in the early 1980s, to make up for those who missed education opportunities during the Cultural Revolution, its focus since the mid-1980s contributed more to the creation of two higher education systems in China. This strategy also turned out to be harming the reputation of adult higher education. In early years adult higher education was a pioneer and well supported politically. Following the massification of higher education, however, it came to be seen as second rate and responsible for a perceived lowering of standards. All the applicants who applied for the admission invariably were admitted and thus resulted in a constant lowering of the minimum admission score of degree programs in adult higher education (Li, 2005).

Thus, adult higher education in China could boast its larger enrollment, but not its quality of teaching and learning. Even during its peak, very few universities developed a considerable number of stable teaching and administrative staff to look after the program management and curricular development. In addition, adult higher education institutions did not make sufficient efforts to develop different teaching methods and materials for adult students.

Adult higher education programs could be divided into three groups: face-to-face instruction, distance learning, and self-study. The first type includes two formats—face-to-face full-time teaching modes mainly conducted for secondary school graduates, and part-time face-to-face teaching modes mainly for working adults through evening schools. The second model has a different way of carrying out instruction, either through correspondence, or by radio or television, or online. The third form follows study guidelines and learning materials provided before participating in the national self-study higher education examinations.

Adult higher education programs train a large number of students by "borrowing" teachers from regular higher education. Existing teaching forces from faculties in regular higher education institutions contribute to almost all teaching in adult degree programs. They are given extra financial incentives to deliver teaching in adult higher education programs, provided teaching resources for radio and television universities, and offered some preparatory courses for students taking the self-study higher education examinations by charging them tuition fees. Adult higher education also tends to duplicate some subjects offered in universities. Even though teachers in adult higher education programs make changes in the teaching content for part-time students in order to better fit their studying mode, they usually copy all teaching materials from on-campus full-time undergraduate students for the following reasons.

The Ministry of Education in China used to play a key role in curriculum decisions and was given the power of regulating national teaching plans, outlines, and even textbooks. Government agencies were the designers, coordinators and supervisors of college curriculum development (Wang, 1994). The process of curricular decision-making was characterized as a top-down approach with little participation from universities. After the open-door policy remarkable changes made in the higher education curriculum have clearly geared much teaching toward economic modernization needs (Hayhoe, 1989), but decision-making was left basically unchanged owing to fears that loosing control of curricular content might lead to political instability. Only seven leading universities in China, including Tsinghua University, Peking University and Zhejiang University were given authority to set up their own disciplines for undergraduate programs in 2002. Curricular decision-making structures also confined adult higher education to the development of professional programs to meet market needs. It was also supposed to weather the social and economic environment and to strengthen ties between universities and society.

Even though there were no obvious distinction of teaching content between students in regular institutions of higher education and students in adult institutions of higher education, a huge difference existed in the quality of teaching and learning between two groups of students. China's adult higher education was primarily related to university degree programs. But students in adult higher education programs were granted different certificates to distinguish them from students in regular higher education institutions. This helped to generate the people's perception that adult higher education was not comparable in quality and students are not as competent. As a result, regular higher education institutions in general would not normally assign the most brilliant faculty members to teach in adult higher education programs, and the outlook for employment by adult higher education degree holders was usually not promising since they were considered inferior to regular university degree holders. Students in adult higher education programs therefore often did not possess high motivation to study hard because they did not feel that it would pay off. It was therefore very evident that the policy of differentiating these two qualifications caused serious consequences. Recently, wide-spread scandal and corruption in adult higher education was reported (Li, 2005). This included the leaking of exam content by teachers, cheating in exams by hiring agents to substitute the examinees, faking certificates, and bribing teachers and administers to buy exam papers in advance.

Adult higher education, nevertheless, pioneered and promoted reform in China's once highly centralized higher education. It was adult higher education that first departed from the three-decade long practice of free higher education for all, and introduced stronger links between education and student demands. However, adult higher education with a focus on degree programs could only be developed rapidly in a specific historical period. This was a phenomenon that could not be, and would not be possible, to maintain for a long time.

STRATEGIES OF REFORMING ADULT HIGHER EDUCATION

When the clock turned to the new millennium, it became urgent to find a new direction to develop adult and continuing education for many universities in China. As with other reforms, educational changes were often stimulated by some perceived internal or external crises. The rapid expansion of higher education in China accelerated the crisis in adult and continuing education. The two-decade market-driven reform in China laid a strong foundation for educational restructuring. This also created the huge demand for higher level professional talent in the human capital market.

For decades, the various forms of adult higher education in almost all universities took degree level education as their main undertaking, while often neglecting other types of in-service training in specific skills and continuing education. This phenomenon had two negative impacts. First, the potential problem of low quality in adult higher education was shadowed by the phenomenon of high market demand for certificates. Second, adult education in the universities was not prepared to develop programs of professional continuing education that were related to new disciplines, new techniques and new knowledge in which universities should have potential.

The restructuring of adult higher education became imperative after the rapid growth of enrollment in China's regular higher education institutions. This changing reality forced universities to reconsider the focus of their adult higher education programs. Restructuring centered on changing the direction of adult higher education to provide professional training to upgrade the managerial ability and technical skills of professionals. Also, increasing importance was attached to the provision of professional training for all types of managers. Not only did this change provide a new opportunity to expand the sector, but this also had implications for, and impact on, the adult higher education system, institutional structure, business operation, and program development.

The new strategies adopted by China's universities to restructure adult education were designed to operate under market mechanisms with more authority and flexibility to provide programs that meet the needs of the market. This change in China's adult and continuing education was examined with special reference to the experience in three leading universities in China—Tsinghua University in Beijing, Zhejiang University in Hangzhou, and Sun Yet-san University in Guangzhou. These three higher education institutions have carried out the restructuring of adult and continuing education sector over the last five years. And they are also geographically spread over from China's north and east, to south, and three cities where the universities are located are prosperous commercial metropolis with booming economy.

Restructuring the Adult Higher Education System

The first type of strategy of responses adopted by Chinese universities was to restructuring the adult higher education system. The massification of higher education provided an opportunity to revamp the adult higher education system, and it was developed into much broader areas to incorporate online education, and include continuing professional education.

Adult higher education was traditionally considered as a university extension by offering degree programs to working adults. Historically, this was the most important part of the adult higher education system. Most universities set up a school of adult education in the late 1980s and early 1990s to coordinate all award-bearing programs for working adults. Although the main objectives of adult education were aimed at providing working adults with higher education opportunities in a part-time mode, many universities' adult education also enrolled secondary school graduates failed in the national college entrance examination in a full-time mode. While the latter operation was completed terminated in seventy-six universities under the Ministry of Education in 2006, adult education sector continues to offer part-time degree programs to working adults. And some schools of adult education even established the Academy of Self-study Examination to offer preparatory courses for students taking the self-study higher education examinations. China claimed to have built the largest self-study higher education system in the world, which allowed adult students to complete their postsecondary studies by following the study outline provided by the examination authority. The flexibility of the system permitted adult students to conduct the study in spare time at their own pace.

Online education—once an independent unit in China's higher education system—was put under the umbrella of adult education, and the merger intended to strengthen its role to offer academic degree programs off-campus. Since adult education institutions were allowed to only enroll part-time students, online programs offered in a full-time mode could supplement the traditional adult education by providing a hybrid study mode. The combination of part-time face-to-face teaching and full-time online learning did not violate the government's policy of limiting adult education institutions from offering full-time academic programs. And even more importantly, this approach increased the meeting times between teachers and students both face-to-face and online, thus delivering better teaching outcomes.

Started in 1999 when 67 universities were given a green light to launch programs online, online education enrolled over one million students annually. The programs offered by online education ranged from a higher diploma, to a two-year top-up bachelor degree for those who already had a higher diploma, to a four-year university degree, and to postgraduate courses. Differed from other academic programs, universities were given autonomy to admit students for online programs based on their own criteria, set up the subjects without seeking an approval from the Ministry of Education, decide the tuition fees with more flexibility, grant awards which usually need to be authorized by the Ministry of Education, and allow students to accumulate their credits in a certain period. These factors are attributed to high-speed development of online education, which has become one major area for further expansion of the university's adult education sector.

However, the prime area for expansion and growth was continuing professional education, which became an engine for the further development of adult higher education. Continuing professional education did not start until the late 1980s when the development of the economy required more seasoned managers to run the growing business and professional operation for almost all specializations. Although China has made impressive gains in human resource development after more than two decades into the reform of market economy, the nation is still facing a critical shortage of well-trained managers and professionals. One major reason behind the scarcity of human resources was attributed to the fact that the investment in human capital in China was even below the average of most developing countries such as India, Thailand, Brazil, and Mexico (Heckman, 2002). However, market-driven economic reforms could provide people with incentives to invest in human capital, since talented professionals could move freely around in the labor market with the opportunity of better salary and promotion.

Tsinghua University in Beijing provides the most prominent example in developing continuing professional education programs. Tsinghua started to operate China's first school of continuing education in 1986. In the period of four years since Tisnghua launched the reform in 2003 to focus on continuing professional and executive programs as the core operation of adult education, more than half a million participants have attended various professional development programs offered by the School, and its annual tuition income reached over RMB 400 million in 2007. Tsinghua's continuing education sector has also grown much larger in size since 2003, and the total number of staff members has increased more than ten folds from 2003 to 2007. The development in this area also became a phenomenon nationwide—with rapidly expansion of continuing professional education programs this sector generated additional tuition fees for universities. Thus, it was imperative to establish a business-oriented organization to meet this change, and the purpose of organizational restructuring was aimed at moving aggressively towards corporate management structures.

Establishing a Business-Oriented Organization

The second type of strategy of responses adopted by Chinese universities was to establish a business-oriented organization to implement a corporate-style management. With the arrival of the "Customer Century" in higher education, the university's adult education sector looked into its existing management and reengineered its structure to fit the new changing environment.

A flat center-based structure was promoted and set up along the lines of professional business management to support its reformed operation. The center-based operation was streamlined in line with the practice of the business community. Tsinghua University's School of Continuing Education stated its reform in 2003 to stop degree programs for adults and only run professional development programs, and by Spring 2008 the School had fifteen business centers. At Zhejiang University's School of Adult Education, ten centers were established after its restructuring in 2007 to focus on training for the different profession, trade and industry, while traditional adult education and online education to offer academic degree programs continued to operate. Three centers were formed at Sun Yet-san University's School of Higher Adult Education to specialize on academic programs for adult students, online education, and professional development programs. Though different universities had adopted various approaches, the operation in general tended to be more program-based than department-based, and a head was usually appointed to lead one or two programs with a high-degree of autonomy and flexibility. This eliminated unnecessary layers between the top management and front lines, allowing greater flexibility to react to changes in a timely and effective manner.

The adult higher education sector even established a training center in partnership with private companies for the purpose of seeking financial back-up for the operation. The primary consideration for the collaboration was the lack of funding from the university. But this has broad implication—this type of university-industry alliance would enable the adult education sector to link the educational service with the market closely and even help to introduce corporate governance into its operations. At Tsinghua University, the Center for Professional Training in the Science Park, financially supported by the Science Park adjacent to Tsinghua University, focused on providing training in the areas of marketing and business management, finance, and engineering management for all-level executives in the Park. At Zhejiang University, the Center for IT Training was set up with both the technical and financial support from an IT company to provide training on computer software. At Sun Yet-san University, the program on hotel and hospitality management was launched together with a multinational hotel group for the purpose of internship and placement.

This newly established flat center-based structure provided flexibility and accountability in order to maintain a balance between the transfer of authority and responsibilities. Thus, the devolved budgeting system was implemented so that program teams could make sound decisions in the self-funding operation. Each business unit was a program center which provided different kinds of professional development programs for the specialized fields. It also functioned as a budget unit which was responsible for its own financial outcome and generating sufficient revenue to sustain its own growth.

However, the center-based structure did accelerate bitter competition among the different units. By bringing down the pyramid structure, there was still a need to enhance the horizontal and cross-functional structure in order to promote cooperation between teams to help reduce the internal power struggles and isolation, thus accountability could prevail. Lack of internal integration has also taken a toll with many program teams fighting for resources and territory in three universities. To resolve the internal competition, more trade-or-industry-based centers, instead of discipline-or-specialization-based centers, had been formed to draw a much clearer territory and reduce the possible inner conflict among the centers. The center-based structure not only impeded the horizontal integration, but also obstructed the flow of communications.

Introduction of market mechanisms, which was regarded as a major theme of policy in the management of educational change, brought a fundamental transformation in the structures and management of China's adult and continuing education institutions. The business-oriented operation helped to secure the financial wellbeing of the sector, but more importantly, this transformation bred new values and cultures in China's adult and continuing educational institutions. There was little doubt that the center-based corporate-style structures gave staff much more freedom than they ever had before. The empowerment of employees became a common structural and cultural characteristic of entrepreneurial education organizations. In last two decades, we witnessed the new trend of management, which advocates flexible, self-organizing structures to better respond to the increasing speed of change. The most important qualities for the members of an organization to pursue were those of flexibility and innovation in order to stay in touch with the changing environment, survive and thrive. Thus, the reform and change of the management style opened a new chapter for the organization with the market demands and needs taking a more and more salient position in the outlook of the significant decision makers.

Designing Market-Driven Programs

The third strategy adopted by Chinese universities was to offer more flexible and relevant curricula to meet the changing needs of students and the society. With the introduction of the center-based structure and the underpinning of the entrepreneurial culture, program teams at the adult higher education sector were empowered to look into the opportunity and work with academics and professionals to develop the most needed courses. At the institutional level, the university's adult education sector was given more authority to launch both continuing professional education and online academic programs. They were required to form an academic committee to be responsible for curriculum development, which functioned as an advisory board to make academic decisions.

With the fiercely competitive environment in China's adult higher education sector, universities were required to reverse the traditional way of developing courses. It should have started from feeding information about the learner needs back to the top management then developing and adjusting programs according to the identified needs and wants. Thus, the designing of market-oriented and outcome-based curricula was crucial in the process of successfully launching adult higher education programs demanded by the market. While various channels of developing programs were employed, three approaches were considered as the most important to capitalize on following three kinds of resources—academic staff in the university, experts in the professional bodies, and international cooperation.

The sector attempted to act proactively to the market needs and to closely link the university with the business community. Researchers for program development kept abreast of the changing environment for professional training, and fed back information about market demands through periodical surveys. With the support from the university's academic staff in the program and curriculum design, the adult and continuing education sector quickly introduced high quality programs. By giving sincere consideration of the needs from the perspectives of the business community, authoritative experts in the related field not only included the latest research results in China and abroad, but also integrated theory and practice with a focus on practical application, when designing the curriculum of such programs.

The launch of two programs at Tsinghua University—Auto Marketing and Real Estate Marketing—exemplified the success of this measure. No other sectors in recent years contributed to China's fast growth more than real estate and automobiles. With the booming of these two sectors, the demands for specialized marketing professionals rose sharply. When the opportunity was noticed, the program teams mobilized all resources, working with the academic staff in the university and business leaders in these two sectors, and launched the programs in 2003 in the three most developed cities in China—Beijing, Shanghai, and Guangzhou. Some prominent Professors in management and marketing from the universities taught the programs, and CEOs from the top car makers and the big real estate developers in China were invited to deliver guest lectures.

The second common approach used in launching the market-oriented programs was to utilize the knowledge of experts in the field and the professional bodies, since they understood the trends in the field and the market needs. The school kept direct communication channels with the training departments of some professional bodies, and even involved them in designing the programs. Zhejiang University, for example, launched a program for marketing managers in the silk garment industry together with the Association of

Silk Industry of Zhejiang Province. This type of collaboration and alliance became a common approach in the adult and continuing education sector. At Sun Yet-san University, the hotel and hospitality management program was launched together with a multinational hotel group. This strategic alliance, thus, transformed elite universities with a disassociation from market needs to be more responsive to the pulse of the market.

International partnership was the third approach to offer adult and continuing education programs. International cooperation was an important aspect of educational development in China. During the twentieth century Chinese educators encountered varied foreign influences and became more proactive in utilizing them to pioneer their own national path toward educational development (Ding, 2001). The impact of globalization in China has served as a very important way to provide the professionals with better learning opportunities. International partners include some leading universities and professional bodies worldwide. Almost all cooperative programs with overseas partners had one thing in common: the adult and continuing education sector was unable to locate experts in China to help it develop, or was not allowed to develop due to the government regulation.

In general, the adult and continuing education institutions in China were not permitted to launch postgraduate level programs. At Sun Yet-san University in Guangzhou, the School of Higher Adult Education decided to set up the Joint Center for Professional Training with the University of Hong Kong's School of Professional and Continuing Education (HKU SPACE). The Center has recruited more than 500 students for two postgraduate diploma programs offered by HKU SAPCE. At Tsinghua University in Beijing, the Center for International Collaboration was established to develop professional master's degree programs with overseas universities as the key partners. In China, a large number of higher diploma or bachelor degree holders were keen to receive further education and wished to be enrolled in the professional master degree programs in order to gain competence to be able to compete in the job market. But the postgraduate programs in China's higher education system tended to be more research oriented. Such a vacuum provided a great opportunity for continuing education to meet the market demand. In just less than three years, the Center developed twenty-five executive programs which could top-up to overseas professional master degree programs.

In developing continuing professional education programs, it clearly showed that adult higher education institutions involved more experts in various professional bodies and associations than academics. And the content of programs was strongly influenced by professional bodies and job market (Henkel and Kogan, 1988). As a result, there were better interrelations between theory and application in the program designed for professional adult students. Responsiveness to the market needs and better marketing and communicating with learners were the key to the success of adult and continuing education. However, only quality in the end helped to establish an enduring reputation of an educational institution and attract more potential learners.

Developing Customer-Oriented Quality Assurance

Assuring high quality of professional programs was the forth strategy of response adopted by universities in China in restructuring the adult and continuing education sector. This is a very important step in the process of market-driven program development and management. It is, however, not an easy task to define quality. While people in the educational organization agree with the importance of academic quality, in practice it is always debatable on how to define it and achieve it, since the school, teachers, and students may have had the different criteria for assessing quality. However, it has been found to be particularly true that in continuing education organizations "quality is meeting or exceeding student expectations" (Lumby, 2001, p. 70).

Quality assurance included two aspects. One was the academic aspect, including content and design. The other was the administrative aspect. The restructuring of continuing education in China has provided an unprecedented opportunity to change people's perceptions. At Tsinghua University, the School of Continuing Education has adopted the market-oriented approach in pursuit of quality assurance, which can be viewed as a new form of legitimizing continuing education. This drive towards quality assurance "can be seen partly as a strategy to secure market share and partly as a means to elevate the status of and generate confidence in the sector" (Cheung and Pyvis, 2006).

In the academic facet, the School set up the Department of Academic Management, in order to systematize the procedure of launching new programs, and supervised teaching quality and evaluation. Programs teams were required to do the following before any programs could be launched. Firstly, to submit the program document to the department; secondly, to set up the Validation Panel comprised of the experts in both the academic and professional fields, to make sure that the program was well-designed and ready to be launched; thirdly, the program needed to be approved by the Administrative Office of Professional Training before advertised. However, the quality assurance mechanism was still in the infant stage, and was not systematically implemented across all the programs. Differing from the full-time on-campus academic programs, the approach to quality in the School tended to center on students or other customers. "The market-led system will generate consumer oriented approaches to quality assessment" (Barnett, 1992, p. 3). The School considered feedback given by learners in evaluating program quality as very important and highly valued comments given by industry professionals in evaluating program quality.

The rapid growth of executive and professional programs might come at the cost of lowered quality. Therefore, a new mechanism of quality review must be established along with the restructuring of continuing education. Hong Kong's experience shows that quality assurance measures of parent universities, if applied strictly in vetting continuing education courses, have been found to be too stringent and inflexible (Cheng and Pyvis, 2006). The continuing education sector in Hong Kong has set up its own quality assurance mechanisms. Thus, continuing education institutions in China should be encouraged to channel more resources into ensuring quality. While the market-oriented and learner-oriented approach may be considered to be the primary and the most important way to assure quality in adult and continuing education, the professional evaluation, accreditation and peer review should also be included to maintain appropriate balance.

Regarding the administrative aspect, three universities—Tsinghua, Zhejiang, and Sun Yat-san—were quite exemplary, particularly impressive in their efforts to provide administrative support and service to learners. The ways in which students were supported and served illustrated their intention to ensure that good teaching and learning environment were provided. In general, one administrative staff in the program team was assigned to take care of each cohort and was responsible for students' overall needs. This not only covered the activities in the academic side, and requests for classroom support, but also included accommodations and hotel arrangements. By demonstrating high standards of quality for teaching and student support services that cut across the whole institution, these three universities were able to communicate effectively about their strengths with students, prospects, and other stakeholders.

In a sense the adult and continuing education sector in China has adopted the measures of total quality management, which have been advocated in the private business for many years and have also in recent years been embraced in the public sector of the West to assure quality services. As program leaders, they were judged on the basis of the quality of programs they supervised and the revenue they generated for their schools. The importance of market orientation was attached to the program development and management from program planning and packaging to student admission and teaching arrangements. Each program team needed to respond proactively to the market demand. This outcome-oriented culture reshaped the organizational fabric of China's adult and continuing education.

This global trend of marketization has been identified as "academic capitalization" in the university sector (Slaughter and Leslie, 1997). Its impact on China's adult and continuing education has fundamentally changed the tradition of educational institutions. The ways of developing programs are very much market-oriented, while various channels have been employed to market the programs to professionals. Even quality assurance mechanism has shifted its focus from peer review to student-centered evaluation. Thus, such a new culture has been stimulated and reinforced as a result of this transformation.

Discussion and Conclusion

Change usually is evaluated with regard to its desirability and feasibility. To discuss the desirability of repositioning adult higher education, it is necessary to understand why the old way of running adult college degree programs could not be sustained any longer. In its early years adult higher education provided opportunities for adults to attain higher education in China. Following the policy of massive expansion of higher education in recent years, however, the changing environment in the market of adult higher education left no better alternative than a fundamental reform of the system itself. Thus, this policy change and internal crisis triggered many adult higher education institutions in China to begin their repositioning in order to survive in the new environment.

To discuss the feasibility of launching such reform, it is clear that the global change from an over-centralized economic planning model to the one which combines state planning and market force regulation has led to greater autonomy in the decision-making of higher education. It is also apparent that the ongoing process of economic reform in China has created a wholly new human capital market. The increasing demands for professional talent have generated the possibility for the adult higher education sector to steer a new course. This is in the direction of professional training instead of focusing only on academic degree programs for adults. In addition, the global trend towards marketization in higher education has provided a foundation for policy cross-fertilization and selective adoption in implementing such reforms in China's adult higher education sector.

The way of responding to challenges by Chinese universities has noticeably demonstrated that market forces have been introduced as the major influence in China's adult higher education. The introduction of market-like relationships to achieve institutional efficiency has been adopted in the process of revamping the system and structure. The adult higher education sector has been reshaped by the application of corporate governance in its internal management and the emphasis on market needs in launching professional development programs. "The idea of the university as a community of scholars, students or disciplines, and as a public agency to some extent yielded to the idea of the university as a corporate enterprise" (Bleiklie, 2002, p. 30). This transformation has dual effects. First, it has helped the university's adult education to proactively respond to the needs of the market. Second, it has fundamentally changed the way that traditional universities functioned and "performativity" has become the norm.

The restructuring of China's adult and continuing education has clear purposes. The state needs to ensure that some types of educational institutions can survive and expand without government funding by decentralizing and devolving more autonomy to them. In the restructuring of adult and continuing education, it is hoped that the state would not need to fund the sector of lifelong learning, and that adult and continuing education could be tied more closely to relevant economic policy and perceived labor market needs. As such, it could be strongly argued that restructuring of adult and continuing education in these aspects are strategic moves rather than instrumental measures.

As a result of the transformation of the centrally planned economy into the socialist market economy, the Chinese government desires to release its control on areas that are not strategically significant. The move of decentralizing this particular area of professional education indeed demonstrates that the state is willing to loosen up its direct control in the area in which the ideological influence is not regarded as so important as in primary, secondary, and even postsecondary education. The government also intends to demonstrate in the process of this reform that public institutions, such as education, can rely less on financial support from the government. By restructuring the adult and continuing education sector, it may help to accumulate valuable experience for a larger scale reform in higher education.

As in many other countries, China no longer considers that human capital development should be solely the responsibility of the government, and market forces are replacing state forces as the major driving forces for the development of adult and continuing education. As a result, adult and continuing education has become a consumption item, and adult and continuing education institutions are the suppliers in the market which aim to meet market demands for manpower training. This market-driven approach to adult education and training is concerned mainly with developing the economy (Walters, 2000). Therefore, the strategies adopted by university's adult and continuing education in China in restructuring this sector have been consistent with the global trend of marketization in higher education.

However, the restructuring of China's continuing education should not solely consider the needs of executive and professional training. Apple (1999) strongly rejects any approach that reduces education to mere training or is not grounded in the personal lives and stories of real teachers, students, and community members. Human resource development and lifelong learning should also contribute to broader educational goals, to critical thinking and to human development more broadly. This may also help to foster the earning capacity of the poor and eventually reduce poverty and enhance welfare while spurring economic growth. The government's priorities should therefore include improvements to the general equity, efficiency, and quality of education (Hossain, 1997). Thus, adult and continuing education should not only respond to market demands, but also devote its efforts to serving a wide array of social functions and values. The balance between adult and continuing education as a social institution and as a self-funding business entity should be maintained to resist complete adaptation to corporate values in adult and continuing education.

REFERENCES

Agelasto, M., and Adamson, B. (Eds.). (1998). *Higher education in post-Mao China.* Hong Kong: Hong Kong University Press.

Apple, M. W. (1999). *Power, meaning, and identity.* New York: Peter Lang.

Apple, M. W. (2001). Comparing neo-liberal projects and inequality in education. *Comparative Education, 37* (4), 409-423.

Baldwin, G., and James, R. (2000). The market in Australian higher education and the concept of student as informed consumer. *Journal of Higher Education Policy and Management, 22* (2), 139-148.

Barnett, R. (1992). *Improving higher education: Total quality care.* Berkshire, UK: SRHE and Open University Press.

Bie, Dunrong (1999). Managing universities autonomously in China. *Journal of Higher Education, 20* (5), 29-31.

Blaug, M. (1970). *Education vouchers, economics of education.* Harmondsworth: Penguin.

Bleiklie, I. (2002). Explaining change in higher education policy. In P. R. Trowler (Ed.), *Higher education policy and institutional change* (pp. 24-45). Buckingham: SRHE and Open University Press.

Bridges, D. (1994). Parents: Customers or partners?. In D. Bridges and T. H. McLaughlin (Eds.), *Education and the market place* (pp. 1-8). London: Falmer Press.

Campbell, J. L., and Peterson, O. K. (2001). *The rise of neoliberalism and institutional analysis.* Princeton, New Jersey: Princeton University Press.

CCPCC and State Council (1993). *The outline for reform and development of education in China.* Beijing: The Chinese Communist Party Central Committee and the State Council.

CCPCC and State Council (1998). *Decision on deepening educational reforms and comprehensively promoting quality-oriented education.* Beijing: The Chinese Communist Party Central Committee and the State Council.

Cheung, C., and Pyvis, D. (2006). How university-based adult continuing education organizations have responded to Hong Kong's changing educational needs since the 1997 transfer of sovereignty. *Research in Post-Compulsory Education, 11* (2), 153-173.

China Education Yearbook 1949-1981 (1984). Beijing: China Encyclopaedia Press.

Clark, B. R. (1998). *Creating entrepreneurial universities: Organizational pathways of transformation.* Oxford: Pergamon.

Currie, J. (1998). *Impact of globalization on Australian universities: Competition, fragmentation and demoralization.* Paper presented at International Sociology Association World Congress.

Ding, Gang (2001). Nationalization and internationalization: Two turning points in China's education in the twentieth century. In G. Peterson, R. Hayhoe and Y. L. Lu (Eds.), *Education, culture, and identity in twentieth-century China* (pp. 161-186). Hong Kong: Hong Kong University Press.

Evans, P., Rusechemeyer, D., and Skocpol, T. (1985). *Bringing the state back in*. Cambridge: Cambridge University Press.

Green, A. (1997). *Education, globalization and the nation state*. London: Macmillan.

Hayhoe, R. (1989). *China's universities and the open door*. New York: Sharp.

Hayhoe, R. (Ed.). (1992). *Education and modernization: The Chinese experience*. Oxford: Pergamon.

Heckman, J. J. (2002). *China's investment in human capital.* National Bureau of Economic Research Working Paper Series.

Henkel, M., and Kogan, M. (1988). Changes in curriculum and institutional structures: Responses to outside influences in higher education institutions. In C. Gellert (Ed.), *Innovation and adaptation in higher education* (pp. 66-91). London: Jessica Kingsley.

Hossain, Shaikh I. (1997). Making education in China equitable and efficient. *World Bank Policy Research Paper Series, No. 1814.*

Kandel, I. L. (1933). *Studies in comparative education.* Boston: Houghton Mifflin.

Kenway, J. (1992). *Marketing education in the post-modern age*. Paper presented at the AARE Conference San Francisco.

Kwiek, M. (Ed.). (2003). The state, the market, and higher education: Challenges for the new century. In M. Kwiek (Ed.), *The university, globalization, central Europe* (pp. 71-114). New York: Peter Lang.

Lauder, H., and Hughes, D. (1999). *Trading in futures: Why markets in education don't work.* Philadelphia: Open University Press.

Li, Xiaoping (2000). University autonomy in China - history, present situation and perspective. In OECD (Ed.), *Current issues in Chinese higher education* (pp. 37-42). Paris: OECD.

Li, Yang (2005, December 19-25). The fall of adult education. *China Newsweek, 257*, 22-24.

Lumby, J. (2001). *Managing further education: Learning enterprise*. London: Paul Chapman.

MoE (1998). *Action plan to revitalize education towards the twenty-first century*. Beijing.

Mok, K. H. (2002). Policy of decentralization and changing governance of higher education in post-Mao China. *Public Administration and Development, 22* (3), 261-273.

Naughton, B. (1995). *Growing out of the plan*. Cambridge: Cambridge University Press.

Ngok, K. L., and Kwong, J. (2003). Globalization and educational restructuring in China. In K. H. Mok and A. Welch (Eds.), *Globalization and educational restructuring in the Asia Pacific Region* (pp. 160-188). New York: Palgrave Macmillam.

Olssen, M., and Peters, M. A. (2005). Neoliberalism, higher education and the knowledge economy: From the free market to knowledge capitalism. *Journal of Education Policy, 20* (3), 313-345.

Postiglione, G. (2003). Universities for knowledge economies: Hong Kong and the Chinese Mainland within globalization and decentralization. In K. H. Mok (Ed.), *Centralization and decentralization: Educational reforms and changing governance in Chinese societies* (pp. 157-172). Hong Kong: The University of Hong Kong.

Slaughter, S., and Leslie, L. L. (1997). *Academic capitalism*. Baltimore, MD: The Johns Hopkins University Press.

State Council (1987). *Decision on development and reform of adult education*. Beijing.

Thomas, R. M. (1983). *Politics and education: Cases from eleven nations*. New York: Pergamon Press.

Tiffin, J., and Rajasingham, L. (1995). *In search of the virtual class education in an information society*. London: Rutledge.

Walters, S. (2000). Globalization, adult education, and development. In N. P. Stromquist and K. Monkman (Eds.), *Globalization and education: Integration and contestation across cultures* (pp. 197-218). Lanham, MD: Rowman and Littlefield.

Wang, Jing (1994). *Curriculum decision making in Chinese higher education*. Unpublished PhD Dissertation, State University of New York, Albany.

Wang, X. (2001). A policy analysis of the financing of higher education in China: Two decades reviewed. *Journal of Higher Education Policy and Management, 23* (2), 205-217.

Whitty, G.., Power, S., and Halpin, D. (1998). *Devolution and choice in education*. Philadelphia: Open University Press.

Yin, Q., and White, G. (1994). The marketization of Chinese higher education: A critical assessment. *Comparative Education, 30* (3), 217-237.

In: New Research in Education Adult, Medical and Vocational ISBN 978-1-60741-873-3
Editors: Edmondo Balistrieri and Giustino DeNino © 2009 Nova Science Publishers, Inc.

Chapter 3

MINIMIZING THE IMPACT OF WRITTEN SCREENING TOOLS ON THE MANAGEMENT OF ADULT PATIENTS WITH LOW HEALTH LITERACY

Timothy V. Johnson and Viraj A. Master
Department of Urology
Emory University School of Medicine, Altanta, GA, USA

Sir William Osler, the 'Father of Modern Medicine,' said "If you listen carefully to the patient, he will tell you the diagnosis." Today, physicians face increasing pressure to expedite medical care, often to the detriment of fully listening to the patient. Consequently, physicians use written screening tools to save time and theoretically facilitate communication with the patient. Physicians hope that patients will generate the diagnosis themselves, a 21st century compromise between modern time constraints and Oslerian communication and observation.

However, what if a patient administers a questionnaire inaccurately? We have shown that up to 70% of patients misrepresent their symptoms on common written screening tools. Given the role of screening tools in place of part of the medical interview, these inaccurate scores could influence medical decisions, placing patients with low health literacy at increased risk for inappropriate management, such as unnecessary surgery. Consequently, we designed an electronic screening tool that reduces misunderstanding and improves patient satisfaction. Through this novel use of technology, we have reconciled screening tools with Osler's concept of communication and observation. As a result, patients in our clinic are safer, better managed, and more satisfied.

THE LOW HEALTH LITERACY EPIDEMIC

Low health literacy constitutes a staggering epidemic in America. Health literacy is a patient's ability to obtain, process, and understand basic health information to make appropriate health decisions.[1] Extensive research has assessed the clinical impact of prose and document (written) literacy. Nearly 90 million American adults have inadequate written health literacy.[1, 2] While the average American adult reads below the 9th grade level, 21% of adults read below the 6th grade reading level.[1, 2] Studies have found that 42% of Medicare enrollees with low health literacy could not understand medication directions, 22% could not understand their appointment slips, and 62% could not understand an informed consent form.[1, 2]

Much less research has focused on the numerical aspect of health literacy, also known as numeracy. However, recent studies have begun to address it, suggesting that unlike written health literacy, low numerical literacy is much more prevalent and affects patients with written literacy and high education level. Rothman et al, for example, reported that 77% of their study population had ninth grade or better literacy skills, but only 37% had ninth or better grade math skills, resulting in a significant inability of the patient population to comprehend nutrition labels.[3] Another study reported that 25% of medical students at a prominent university had imperfect numeracy.[4]

The Impact of Low Health Literacy and Numeracy

Low health literacy and numeracy is not merely a phenomenon of prevalence, but instead has significant negative impact on patient outcomes.[3] First, low health literacy impacts access to services. Patients with low health literacy are twice as likely to have never received a pap smear, and almost 1.5 times more likely to have never received a mammogram, influenza vaccine, or pneumococcal vaccine.[6] Studies have found that 42% of Medicare enrollees with low health literacy could not understand medication directions, 22% could not understand their appointment slips, and 62% could not understand an informed consent form.[5] Studies have also shown that both patients at a public county hospital and Medicare enrollees with low health literacy are more likely to be hospitalized compared to patients with adequate health literacy.[4,5] Low health literacy also impacts compliance with medical therapy. Asthmatics with low health literacy have poorer metered dose inhaler technique.[4] Diabetics with low health literacy have poorer glycemic and higher hemoglobin A1C levels. As a result, low written health literacy has been firmly linked to increased costs of healthcare.[1, 3] While the literature is still incomplete, numeracy likely has an even larger impact on healthcare costs, morbidity, and mortality in comparison to written health literacy, given its larger prevalence.

Patient misunderstanding of written screening tools (WSTs) is an understudied consequence of all aspects of low health literacy. Whereas the focus of early 20th century generalists such as Osler was on diagnosis through observation, patient-administered WSTs shift physician attention to management. Due to time constraints, urologists,[4] endocrinologists,[5] psychiatrists,[6] and dermatologists[7] increasingly rely on WSTs to collect valuable information. These tools, however, are typically written at the 10th grade reading level, well above the average American's reading level (8th grade).[3, 8] Consequently, physicians increasingly rely on patients to diagnose themselves using a tool patients cannot understand: hardly Osler's vision of patient communication.

THE AUS-SS AS A MODEL FOR WRITTEN SCREENING TOOLS

Due to this shift of diagnostic burden, we assessed the impact of low health literacy on patient understanding of WSTs.[9, 10] Our model, the American Urological Association Symptom Score (AUA-SS), is the world's predominant WST for Benign Prostatic Hyperplasia (BPH) (Figure 1).[4]Validated in several studies,[4, 11, 12] it is a seven-item tool used to screen for symptoms, chart clinical progress, and predict prognosis for BPH.[13, 14] The AUA-SS is deemed so important that the American Urological Association (AUA) places the AUA-SS as the centerpiece in its BPH guidelines as the last necessary step before therapy, behind only history and physical examination (Figure 2).[15]

However, because the AUA-SS is self-administered, it is only as reliable as a patient's health literacy. A patient who cannot reliably read is likely to misunderstand the AUA-SS, thus jeopardizing the accuracy of his responses. Therefore, we conducted four prospective studies involving fifteen hundred patients interviewed over the last two years at an underprivileged county hospital and an academic university hospital. We assessed the prevalence, risk factors, and the clinical impact of misunderstanding of the AUA-SS.[9, 10]

LOW HEALTH LITERACY DRIVES MISUNDERSTANDING OF THE AUA-SS

Of the 1,500 patients we interviewed, 70% misunderstood at least half of the AUA-SS (≥4 questions).[9, 10] Unfortunately, 60% of patients claimed to understand the AUA-SS fully, but did not.[9] The majority of patients who did not understand the AUA-SS's text, still responded to the AUA-SS. Since the AUA-SS is designed to be self-administered, a physician may not identify low health literacy in such a patient who completes the AUA-SS, thus increasing the risk of symptom mismanagement in these patients.

We also assessed demographic variables to identify drivers of this misunderstanding, including age, race, ethnicity, homelessness, employment, and income. Of these variables, understanding was impacted by only three factors: written health literacy, numeracy, and education level, a surrogate for health literacy. Compared to patients who read at the high school level, patients who read at the elementary school level were *28 times* more likely to misunderstand the AUA-SS.[9] Additionally, patients with low numeracy were also 3.5 times more likely to misunderstand the AUA-SS, independent of education or written health literacy level.

This poorer misunderstanding of the AUA-SS is not only a theoretical deficit, but can be translated to an actual risk to patient care. Once patients self-administer the AUA-SS, their score is categorized into a low, medium, or high severity. These severity categories consequently drive disease management. Patients with low health literacy, numeracy, and education levels miscategorize the severity of their AUA-SS scores twice as often as other patients. Given the AUA-SS's status in the AUA's BPH guidelines as a reliable tool,[4, 11, 12] these findings suggest that patients with low literacy levels are at significant risk of both under- and over-treatment of their symptoms.

Name: Date:

	Not at all	Less than 1 time in 5	Less than half the	About half the time	More than half the	Almost always	Your score
Incomplete emptying Over the past month, how often have you had a sensation of not emptying your bladder completely after you finish urinating?	0	1	2	3	4	5	
Frequency Over the past month, how often have you had to urinate again less than two hours after you finished urinating?	0	1	2	3	4	5	
Intermittency Over the past month, how often have you found you stopped and started again several times when you urinated?	0	1	2	3	4	5	
Urgency Over the last month, how difficult have you found it to postpone urination?	0	1	2	3	4	5	
Weak stream Over the past month, how often have you had a weak urinary stream?	0	1	2	3	4	5	
Straining Over the past month, how often have you had to push or strain to begin urination?	0	1	2	3	4	5	

	None	1 time	2 times	3 times	4 times	5 times or more	Your score
Nocturia Over the past month, many times did you most typically get up to urinate from the time you went to bed until the time you got up in the morning?	0	1	2	3	4	5	

Total IPSS score	

Quality of life due to urinary symptoms	Delighted	Pleased	Mostly satisfied	Mixed – about equally satisfied and dissatisfied	Mostly dissatisfied	Unhappy	Terrible
If you were to spend the rest of your life with your urinary condition the way it is now, how would you feel about that?	0	1	2	3	4	5	6

Total score: 0-7 Mildly symptomatic; 8-19 moderately symptomatic; 20-35 severely symptomatic.

Figure 1. American Urological Association Symptom.

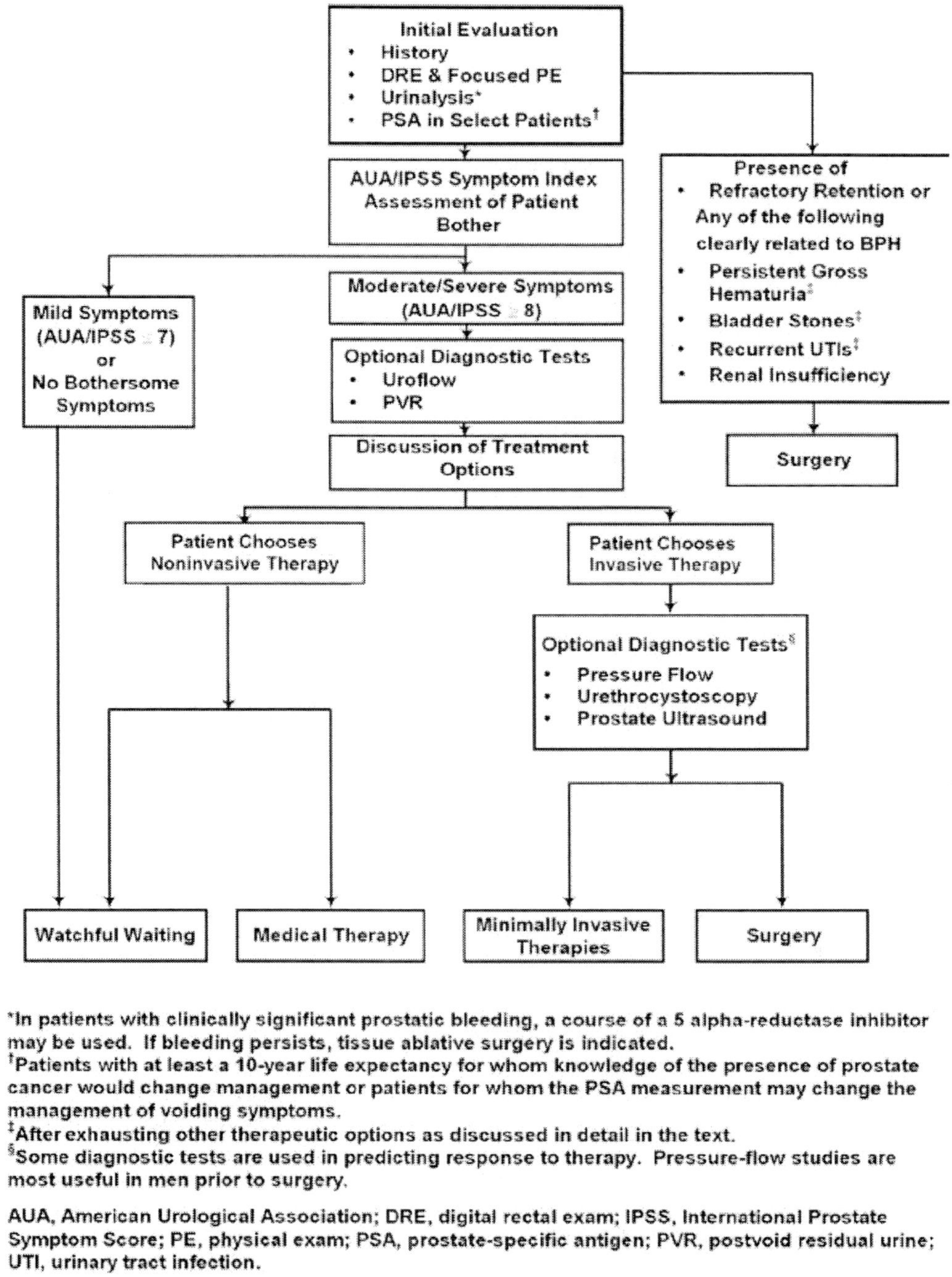

Figure 2. Benign prostatic hyperplasia (BPH) diagnosis and treatment.

COMPUTERIZED SCREENING TOOLS AS THE SOLUTION

Despite poor performance of the AUA-SS, there is cause for optimism: patient understanding depends only on health literacy and education levels. Unlike fixed factors such as age and race, these factors can be overcome. Many studies have attempted to overcome low health literacy. For example, physicians have simplified sentence structure in consent forms.[16] However, there are limits to simplification before meaning is lost.[16] Others have supplemented text with pictures, ideal for short commands.[17] The most effective and widely applicable method for overcoming low health literacy may be multimedia audiovisual instruction.[17]

Therefore, we designed a novel multimedia version of the AUA-SS. This computer program displays the original AUA-SS with explanatory videos that read the questions aloud and teach patients how to select answers properly. We tested the efficacy of the computerized AUA-SS through a randomized clinical trial. We randomized 232 patients, demographically similar to our previous 1,500 patients, to either the traditional AUA-SS or computerized AUA-SS.

Our findings suggest that the computerized AUA-SS cuts misunderstanding by *50%* across all literacy levels. This reduction was unaffected by patient computer familiarity. Moreover, all patients completed the computerized AUA-SS, versus 8% of patients who did not complete the traditional AUA-SS. Finally, patients reported higher satisfaction with the computerized AUA-SS.

Conclusions

The AUA-SS, created to expedite the medical interview, places patients with low health literacy at increased risk of receiving inappropriate care. Osler once said, "The secret of the care of the patient is in caring for the patient." Therefore, we created a computerized version of the AUA-SS. This multimedia questionnaire significantly reduces misunderstanding, thereby minimizing patients' risk of mismanagement and increasing patient satisfaction. This tool allows physicians to expedite the medical interview while preserving the Oslerian principle of communication with patients.

References

[1] Davis TC, W. M.: Health Literacy: Implications for Family Medicine. *Fam Med.,* 36: 595, 2004

[2] Kirsch I, Junglebut A., Jenkins L, Kolstad A: Adult literacy in America: a first look at the findings of the national adult literacy survey. Washington, DC: National Center for Education Statistics, U.S. Department of Education, 1993. Accessed online January 12, 2008, at: http://nces.ed.gov/pubs93/93275.pdf

[3] Safeer RS, K. J.: Health literacy: the gap between physicians and patients. *Am. Fam. Physician.*, 72: 463, 2005

[4] Barry, M. J. F., F J, Jr; O'Leary, M P; Bruskewitz, R C; Holtgrewe, H L; Mebust, W K; Cockett, A T: The American Urological Association symptom index for benign prostatic hyperplasia. The Measurement Committee of the American Urological Association. *Journal of Urology*, 148: 1549, 1992

[5] Schillinger D, G. K., Piette J, Wang F, Osmond D, Daher C, Palacios J, Sullivan GD, Bindman AB.: Association of health literacy with diabetes outcomes. *JAMA*, 288: 475, 2002

[6] Yesavage, J. A., Brink, T. L., Rose, T. L. et al.: Development and validation of a geriatric depression screening scale: a preliminary report. J Psychiatr Res, 17: 37, 1982

[7] Finlay, A. Y., Khan, G. K.: Dermatology Life Quality Index (DLQI)--a simple practical measure for routine clinical use. *Clin. Exp. Dermatol.,* 19: 210, 1994

[8] Davis, T. C., Crouch, M. A., Wills, G. et al.: The gap between patient reading comprehension and the readability of patient education materials. *J. Fam. Pract.*, 31: 533, 1990

[9] Johnson, T. V., Goodman, M., Master, V. A.: The efficacy of written screening tools in an inner city hospital: literacy based limitations on patient access to appropriate care. *J. Urol.*, 178: 623, 2007

[10] Johnson, T., Abbasi, A., Ehrlich, S. et al.: Patient misunderstanding of the individual questions of the American Urological Association Symptom Score. *J. Uro*l, In press., 2008

[11] MacDiarmid SA, G. T., Holmes TM, Martin PR, Doyle RB.: An assessment of the comprehension of the American Urological Association Symptom Index. *J. Urol.*, 159: 873, 1998

[12] Netto Junior NR, d. L. M.: The influence of patient education level on the International Prostatic Symptom Score. *J. Urol.*, 154: 97, 1995

[13] Fitzpatrick, J. M.: The natural history of benign prostatic hyperplasia. BJU Int, 97 Suppl 2: 3, 2006

[14] Lukacs, B., Grange, J. C., Comet, D.: One-year follow-up of 2829 patients with moderate to severe lower urinary tract symptoms treated with alfuzosin in general practice according to AUA-SS and a health-related quality-of-life questionnaire. BPM Group in General Practice. *Urology*, 55: 540, 2000

[15] Kaplan, S. A.: Update on the american urological association guidelines for the treatment of benign prostatic hyperplasia. *Rev. Urol.*, 8 Suppl 4: S10, 2006

[16] Meade, C. D., Howser, D. M.: Consent forms: how to determine and improve their readability. *Oncol. Nurs Forum*, 19: 1523, 1992

[17] Communicating with patients who have limited literacy skills. Report of the National Work Group on Literacy and Health. *J. Fam. Pract.*, 46: 168, 1998

1. Dewalt DA BN, Sheridan S, Lohr KN, Pignone MP. Literacy and health outcomes: a systematic review of the literature. J Gen Intern Med 2004;19:1228-39.
2. Howard DH, Gazmararian J, Parker RM. The impact of low health literacy on the medical costs of Medicare managed care enrollees. The American journal of medicine 2005;118:371-7.
3. Rothman RL, Housam R, Weiss H, et al. Patient understanding of food labels: the role of literacy and numeracy. Am J Prev Med 2006;31:391-8.
4. Sheridan SL, Pignone M. Numeracy and the medical student's ability to interpret data. Eff Clin Pract 2002;5:35-40.

In: New Research in Education Adult, Medical and Vocational ISBN 978-1-60741-873-3
Editors: Edmondo Balistrieri and Giustino DeNino © 2009 Nova Science Publishers, Inc.

Chapter 4

VOCATIONAL EDUCATION AND ECONOMIC DEVELOPMENT: A STUDY OF GHANA

George M. Osei
Mansfield College, University of Oxford, UK

ABSTRACT

The paper explores the promise, problems and pitfalls of vocational forms of secondary schooling when these are set up in developing countries. Taking Ghana as a case study, the author presents empirical evidence to examine some of the assumptions of human capital theory, and concludes that there are important limitations which prevent vocational schools from responding adequately to the requirements for economic development. The reasons for the failure of such innovations need to be identified not only from within the educational institution, but also from the wider macro-economic perspective.

Keywords: Vocationalised curriculum, economic development, human capital theory, tracer study, Ghana

INTRODUCTION

In the past 21- years, the Ghanaian education system has undergone a significant and ambitious reform process. The educational reforms undertaken in this period of time – a process without precedent in recent Ghanaian history – have affected all aspects of the educational system, including the curricula and teachers' careers. The Ghanaian educational system has been made to adapt to modern society's needs and demands, including those of the job market, even as democratic structures and methods have been introduced into the system itself. The 1987 reforms set out to increase access to education at all levels, to improve quality of education, diversify the curriculum by introducing vocational and technical subjects. These changes were conceived to correct an educational system perceived as elitist, and which downgraded vocational and technical education.

Attempts to vocationalise Ghana's educational system have a long history, and go back to at least 1974, when, under the government of Kofi A. Busia, vocational/technical schools were set up as a pilot scheme (Antwi, 1992). Eventually, in 1987 the military regime under Jerry J. Rawlings introduced a vocationalised curriculum in secondary schools as one of the key solutions to Ghana's main economic problem: the almost total absence of an indigenous industrial base. Various vocational/technical courses were launched at different periods both by private and by state entrepreneurs from the 1950s onwards, but most of these initiatives failed to attract and keep students long enough to give them adequate training, and indeed, what was provided was often 'too inappreciably connected with any great industry to be regarded as little more than an artistic branch of education' (Fiah, 1981).

The industrialisation of the nation failed to come about despite the very intensive investment in vocational/technical education in the post-colonial period. But, as has been argued elsewhere (Osei, 2001, 2003, 2004, 2006, 2007, 2009), in a situation of dependence and fragility, only a few alternatives are available to a nation as it attempts to generate a self-sustainable economy, and the belief that education can be a solution to intractable economic problems is often maintained. When the Provisional National Defence Council (PNDC) came into government in 1982, a decision was made to vocationalise one third of the secondary level of schooling through the creation of 'vocational schools'. The new schools were to have 25% of their curriculum dedicated to vocational/technical skills training, and 75% to traditional academic lessons. This was justified, in the face of the opposition's criticisms that general education was being abandoned, by claiming that this was the only way that a solid instruction in vocational skills could be given. In his educational budget speech, Dr Ben-abdallah, the Minister for Education and Culture, insisted that vocational schools would satisfy 'the demand for technical workers and tradesmen which the industrial expansion of our country is aiming for' (Ben-abdallah, 1986).

While the official discourse on vocational schools stressed their economic function, it is clear that these new institutions were to respond to other needs as well. Vocational schools were to help change parents' traditional negative attitude towards vocational/technical education. They would respond to the special education needs of groups of students 'who either show a particular inclination for a trade, or for those who are not particularly keen to follow an academic education' (Daily Graphic, 6 November, 1986). Vocational schools were to help check the serious unemployment problems which plagued Ghana as it tried to restructure its economy. Emergency labour corps had been established to mop up some of the unemployed. However, reluctant school-attenders who found themselves blocked from entry into full-time work had to be offered a palatable alternative to the 'irrelevant' academic schooling then offered, and vocational schools, which promised to reproduce the workshop environment besides continuing with general education, were thought to be attractive to those who were either unable or unwilling to pursue traditional courses of study.

ECONOMIC ASPECTS AND CAREER ASPIRATION

Economic aspects, job aspiration and the curriculum choice of clients seem to be important consideration, such as studies by Foster (1965); King and Martin (2002) in Ghana; Lauglo and Narman (1987), Nishimura and Orodho (1999) in Kenya; Nwakoby and Lewin (1991) in Nigeria, all highlight the close inter-relationship between the demands of the economy (experienced through the job market), and the viability of vocationalisation. In effect, the problem for which vocationalisation is offered as solution, may lie well beyond the boundaries of formal education, an issue which is addressed in the concluding part of the paper.

Both parents and students see education as an avenue for social and economic mobility and invest in the kind of education that is perceived to be appropriate and effective for this purpose. In Ghana, as elsewhere, academic education is perceived to hold this key to success and any other form is unacceptable as being lower in status. Consequently, vocational education stands a very poor chance against the academic. Even where access to academic education is very limited, students would go through vocational courses as a preparation for more effective competition to enter the grammar schools. The modern secondary schools in Ghana in the 1950s and 1960s for example, ended up, as was reported, offering a purely academic course which provides only a superficial polishing of the education received at the primary school. Bacchus (1980) reported a similar practice in Guyana amongst students of non-elite schools where vocational subjects were supposed to be taught: students only go through the course so as to prepare better for later access to what is seen as a more valid form of education.

This represents the realities of the aspirations of school leavers and their parents in terms of occupations and in relation to the curricular offerings of schools. Whereas the goals of vocational education generally may emphasize orientation to jobs in the rural locality, school leavers and their parents, aim at access into the modern sector that offers higher incomes and modern life styles. We address a set of issues that are more pressing, particularly for developing countries: is the current level of secondary vocational/technical education (SVTE) appropriate for the current needs of the economy? Does skills development within vocational schools represent the best available education investment strategy for economic development and growth? How should present provision change in the light of planned growth, technological change and development targets? There are two pertinent issues here. First, in periods of economic change, what balance needs to be struck between alternative forms of schooling (vocational/technical schools as opposed to general, academic schools at the secondary level)? Secondly, what forms of skill preparation (SVTE versus other, non-schooling training modes) serve the economy best, particularly in facilitating industrial growth and development?

Some 40 years ago, P. J. Foster, a sociologist from the University of Chicago, published an article that was to become one of the seminal contributions to the vocational education literature (Foster, 1965). The paper, entitled 'The vocational school fallacy in development planning,' had an immediate impact and it still exerts a major influence on the way we think about this pertinent issue. This economic perception of the students was famously argued by Foster (1965) in relation to Ghana. Refuting the white-collar job syndrome, he asserted that:

The operative fact here is not that graduates [of schools] will not accept certain types of employment but rather that the schools (irrespective of what they teach) have been shrewdly used as the gateway into the 'emergent' sector of the economy. The schools themselves can do little about this. So long as parents and students perceive the function of education in this manner, agricultural education and vocational instruction in the schools is [sic] not likely to have a determinative influence on the occupational aspirations and destinations of students. Aspirations are determined largely by the individual's perception of opportunities within the exchange sector of the economy, destinations by the actual structure of opportunities in that sector. (Foster, 1965, p. 151)

A central argument of that paper was whether or not education is truly 'vocational' depends less on the nature of the particular course of study pursued but rather on its relevance to the job opportunities pertaining in the labour market. The theme was further taken up by Mark Blaug in his classic text on the economics of education, where he discusses the usual distinction between academic and vocational education:

This distinction, which is actually grounded in the nature of the two curricula, is allowed to carry the implication that some education prepares students for the 'world of work' and some does not. All too frequently, however, those who have taken courses of study generally called 'academic' … reap substantial financial returns from their education, thus producing the paradoxical conclusion that academic education has a greater 'vocational' value than vocational education. The traditional distinction was developed by educators, but the labour market has its own way of appraising qualifications. (Blaug, 1970, p. 247)

In any case all economies need manual and technical skills for development. Clearly both aspirations and real economic activity, influence what the students wish to learn. Citing another example, Anderson (1970) described a similar experience in Kenya with the establishment of the 'Jeanes Schools' where the clients became disenchanted because they found the course to be offering 'second class' education which only led back to hard manual labour instead of offering access to the wealth and technical advantages of Western life they saw displayed by Europeans. Basically colonial models of and attitudes to academic progress continue to be deeply embedded in post-colonial educational systems in Africa. These colonial vestiges often militate strongly against the development and implementation of innovative and progressive educational ideas and styles such as vocationalism (Crossley and Tikly, 2004; Mayo, 2004; Mulenga, 2004).

It is now generally accepted that access to better jobs, higher wages, higher social status and living standards seem to lie in higher qualifications, preferably at tertiary level. Attempts at vocationalization are thus continuously being reconstructed by the clients to serve perceived individual economic and social aspirations.

The rise of these vocational institutions at the secondary school level, and their ability to respond to ideological, educational and political goals has been documented in detail in another context (Osei, 2001). What this paper sets out to do is to explore the extent to which these vocational schools have in fact fulfilled the economic function which the PNDC government established for them.

Methodology and Data Sources

In order do this, the paper draws on a wide data bank collected within a 'Vocational Secondary School Research Project' (VSSRP) which the author undertook between 2000 and 2004. Quantitative and qualitative research methods used included a detailed questionnaires with 300 twelve year old vocational/technical secondary school students, a tracer study with 100 ex-students,[1] in-depth interviews with 55 students, 25 teachers and instructors, and 10 industrialists and classroom and staffroom observation in vocational/technical secondary schools. The return rates for each of these sub-groups varied from a low of 63% for the teachers to a high of 98% for the students. Follow-up semi-structured interviews were conducted to seek more in-depth data and to clarify issues which arose during preliminary analysis of the questionnaire data. The interviews, on average, lasted more than an hour. They were tape-recorded and later transcribed. When transcribed, the interviews were read and an initial open coding was performed to generate a list of topics (Emerson et al., 1996).

Year 12 ex-students were targeted. To be eligible for participation, students had to have a younger sibling or close relative in the same school or in a related school. The use of family members to trace students exiting the school system was earlier used by Al-Samarrai and Reilly (2005), albeit that their main family informants were parents. Students were presented with lists of occupations devised by the International Labour Organization (ILO) (1987). Parental, particularly paternal, educational levels can be important determinants of future earnings potential in low-income societies (Al-Samarrai and Reilly, 2005; Vlaardingerbroek et al, 2007). Attitudes towards work tend to form in adolescence and are reflected by educational programme choices (Daehlen, 2005). Asking students about anticipated earnings provides useful insights into their perceptions of the labour market (Vlaardingerbroek, 2001).

The quantitative data is supplemented in some areas by surveys carried out by the Guidance and Counselling Unit of the Ministry of Education and the School Industry Unit. The qualitative dimension of the study is based on the grounded theory approach (Glaser and Strauss, 1967). Other forms of documentary evidence were culled from newspapers, and files held at the Ministry of Education.

Human Capital Theory

The setting up of vocational/technical secondary schools represented the most fundamental effort on the part of the PNDC government to link education to the needs of the economy. That effort must not be divorced from other similar attempts by different governments and sustained through the twentieth and twenty-first century as the economy suffered the vagaries of time, or from attempts which were to be made at a later date and addressed at tertiary education (see Ministry of Information, 1986).

---

[1] A tracer study was carried out with two groups of students. The first group consisted of students who left their vocational school before the completion of their third year in 2000/2001; the second group was made up of those who had left after the completion of their third year in 2000/2001. The intention is to follow the students sampled through their occupational careers for a number of years to come, in order to facilitate an extended study of the same respondents. This longitudinal dimension will generate important data regarding the effects of vocational schooling over a period of time.

All these efforts, past and present, were based on a number of assumptions about the link between education and the economy, assumptions which were articulated in a theoretically sophisticated manner by a series of economists from the 1950s onwards through the formulation of what has come to be known as 'human capital theory'. This refers to a view of education as an industry which generates the desired amounts of functional manpower. Knowledge is considered by the likes of Peter Drucker, B. A. Weisbrod and T. W. Schultz, as the only real capital in modern times, and hence, the development of educated people – in vocational and general terms – is the most important capital formulation, and their number, quality and utilisation the most meaningful index of the wealth-production capacity of a country (Sobel, 1978; Small, 2005; Tignor, 2006).

The implications of such views are clear, namely that 'education will produce an increase in general and in job-specific knowledge which individuals subsequently can apply in an expanding economy both to better utilise new technical developments and to generate innovations. The result will be a marked payoff in terms of increased production yielding greater national wealth, corporate profits, and individual wages' (Violas, 1981). Other related assumptions underlying human capital theory are that individuals choose to invest in education and are rewarded accordingly in the labour market, that skills, attitudes and competencies acquired in education are transferable to the workplace, and that the increasing complexity of the workplace and technology requires a higher level of skills of all workers (Blackmore, 1990; World Bank, 2003).

In Ghana, it has been tempting for governments to assume that economic development cannot come about unless there is a highly and appropriately skilled work force, and that one of the ways of achieving that goal is to have diversified educational system which provides vocational/technical education. That assumption has been constant and practically uncontested. For the post-independence period in particular, and in synchrony with developments in other parts of the world, vocational schooling was considered to be a solution to the needs for the diversification of the economy. A consultant in the human capital tradition, such as Arthur Lewis engaged critically with the American school of thought (Lewis, 1953), but ultimately advised the Ghanaian (and other) governments to invest in vocational/technical education, and to embark on five or seven-year plans to calculate and provide the future manpower and skill requirements (Lewis, 1953; Tignor, 2006). The work of Foster (1965) and of Blaug (1973), Berg (1970), Jencks (1972) and Collins (1979), and later of Psacharopoulos (1987), shattered the confidence in human capital that had hitherto been unchallenged. But as the latter scholar pointed out, 'because of its inherently logical and simplistic appeal, vocationalism will be with us for years to come, and more countries will attempt, in vain, to tune their formal educational systems to the world of work' (Psacharopoulos, 1987).

THE ASSUMPTIONS OF HUMAN CAPITAL THEORY

The main assumptions implicit in human capital theory, and with particular reference to vocational schooling, can be presented in a schematic manner. Each of the following assumptions will then be dealt with individually, with each section drawing upon comparative educational literature and empirical studies related to the Ghanaian context, to evaluate the status of each claim. Briefly then, the economic assumptions on which vocational schools in Ghana were developed state that:

1. Schools are well-placed to provide vocational education.
2. Schools can provide skills required by industry in the future.
3. Vocational students do the work they have been trained for
4. There will be positive rates-of-return for vocational students

1. Schools of Vocational Education

There are many problems associated with the assumption that schools are well-placed to provide vocational education (Foster, 1965; King and Martin, 2002). Vocational schools and tracks are generally much more expensive to run than general schools and tracks (Lauglo, 1987; Moura Castro, 1987; King and Martin, 2002; World Bank, 2003), not only in terms of expenditure on material resources (Psacharopoulos, 1987; Ziderman, 2003), but also because class size has to be kept low for pedagogical and safety reasons (Nye and Hedges, 2001). Given the general expenses involved, adequate allocation by the education budget to maintain vocational schools is often lacking, and this is especially true of many developing countries since most of these started off this form of schooling after receiving funding from international agencies such as the International Monetary Fund (IMF) and the World Bank. Once these sources dried up, they then found themselves unable to keep on providing new and up-to-date machinery, tools, equipment or the in-service up-dating courses for vocational/technical teachers (Tilak, 1988; Ziderman, 2003).

Furthermore, educational institutions, hampered by bureaucratic forms of administration, have generally found it difficult to respond to new needs when these are signalled by the labour market (Bowman, 1988; Hutchful, 2002; Sager, 2008), and are often in an impossible situation having to 'prepare students for labour markets without having any control over labour markets themselves or knowledge of how these markets will develop' (Grubb, 1985).

On the other hand, there is a lot of evidence to suggest that industry can train its workers more efficiently, faster and more cheaply than schools can. Industry is clearly more successful than schools can ever be in the creation of the direct experience of production. In addition to this, the training provided by industry is less costly because the workplace has machinery and personnel already used for production and hence incurs less overheads, while students need not forego earnings because they tend to be already employed, or involved in apprenticeship schemes, in the firm which provides the training. Students who are trained on the job and induced in that work environment are much more likely to choose – and remain in – that job, and to be retrained by their employer who has already invested in them. Commitment by the student and the employer is likely to be higher, because both are paying for the training in their own ways, and both wish to re-coup the investment made (Psacharopoulos, 1987, 1988; Ziderman, 1997; World Bank, 2003).

And employers in most parts of the world have in fact generally recognised that schools are not well equipped to provide vocational education, and expect schools to give a good basic education and social and attitudinal skills rather more than credentials, academic or vocational (Bowles, 1973; Oxenham, 1987; King and Martin, 2002; Mandebele and Ephraim, 2008). Given the complex and changing demands of the workplace, employers increasingly cite literacy, flexibility, good work habits, self-discipline, problem-solving skills, and general knowledge as the key qualities they look for in prospective employees (Oakes, 1986; Semple, 1987; King and McGrath, 2002).

Interestingly, most of the extant literature therefore suggests rather strongly that Grubb's hypothesis that the historical ineffectiveness of vocational education can be at least partly explained by the fact that 'it has attempted to do what schools do worst' (Grubb, 1978). The case study of Ghana under consideration bears out this hypothesis. Ghana's vocational schools have been generally unable to respond to the needs of employers and of a changing labour market. A number of Federation of Industry position papers (1999, 2000, 2002) have criticised the quantity and quality of technically trained tradespersons, and while noting that 'the country's educational system is not expected to provide personnel at all levels tailor made for particular industry … it is certainly expected to provide personnel suitably trained in the basics that form the platform for the various industrial sectors' (FOI, 2000).

Additionally, the Federation has insisted that one of the key obstacles to the development of the economy is the serious skills shortage in the light engineering sector, where Ghana is looking to new, high-tech investment. Schools have been unable to respond to the needs for training in the new skills required (Ghanaian Times, 5 April 1999; Daily Graphic, 9 September 2002). The Federation favours a dual training system of vocational education because in this way, private manufacturing companies can offer modern machinery, up-to-date instruction, and the best learning environment since industry offers, better than any school workshop can, the direct experience of production (Ziderman, 1997; Honny, 1999; World Bank, 2003).

A Skills and Training Needs Survey carried out in June 1999 by the Education and Industry Unit with 200 firms concludes that there is a widespread demand by employers of large, medium and small firms for more 'trainable' people (Ofosuhene, 2000). In other words, employers are looking for personal qualities such as motivation, adaptability, standards of work and sense of responsibility, as well as general education, that is literacy and numeracy, the ability to read and follow simple instructions, convey messages accurately, understand simple diagrams, perform basic calculations, and have knowledge of such matters as wages, health and safety rules, social security, work books and trade unions. While the demand for technification implies the need for an increase of 30% at the vocational school level, an emphasis was placed by several employers on the up-grading of the general level of education of unskilled labour rather than on specialised training, and basic rather than advanced technical knowledge was seen to be more useful because of changing machinery which is increasingly becoming much more highly technological (King, 1990; Ziderman, 1997, 2003). In-depth interviews with twenty employers also revealed that at the levels where vocational school students are employed, it is character traits rather than educational or even skills qualifications that are given priority (King and McGrath, 2002).

Ghana's employers generally expressed themselves dissatisfied with the nature of training offered in vocational/technical schools, wanting more up-to-date instruction to be given by more adequately trained instructors, with students utilising more appropriate equipment. Some employers noted that vocational school curricula were restricted, dealing mainly with basic processes, tools and machinery, and many suggestions were made urging the introduction of various skills-training courses reflecting new directions in production. A report commissioned by one vocational school and prepared by a consultant from Great Britain noted that 'machinery and other training equipment available are obsolete and, in some cases, not even operational in view of the lack of parts and maintenance' (Honny, 1999). Funds to redress this situation are becoming less and less available as financial priority is increasingly being given in the Ghanaian educational budget to the post-secondary educational level.

In any case, according to the Skills and Training Needs Survey, some firms were ready to provide machinery and instructors to vocational/technical schools, most were unwilling to incur the costs of training, even when, in the long term, they were the direct beneficiaries and recouped the investment made in human resource development. A UNIDO report on technical training in Ghana confirms the tendency for industry to rely on the vocational training provided by schools, even when they claim to be unhappy with the result (Ofosuhene, 2000). The report argues that employers must be induced to play their part in industrial training programmes, with personnel being released to train teachers and students, and equipment being made available for use in their firms. They could also help by providing up-dating courses to teaching staff in vocational schools and technical institutes.

Nevertheless, the criticisms which employers have levelled at vocational schools must not be accepted at face value. Some of the issues that have been raised show a lack of understanding of the role of vocational schools at the secondary level on the part of industrialists. Vocational school curricula aim to provide local firms with workers at the operative and basic crafts level, and not with technicians. In addition to this, the Ghanaian industrial set-up is characterised by a large percentage of small firms employing less than twenty workers (ISSER, 2000). Such firms are not likely to offer the training facilities that the UNIDO report recommends. Most firms are also unlikely to require an advanced degree of technical skills.

The insistence since 1987 by the PNDC government that Ghana will be transforming its market orientation towards high technological fields that more sophisticated skills will therefore be required, and that secondary schools should change curricula to aim for such sunrise industries, is problematic. Various studies have suggested rather strongly that the widespread and long-standing belief that an increasingly technological society requires a skilled populace is questionable (Braverman, 1974; Ziderman, 1997; King and McGrath, 2002). Rather, what has been shown is that the increasing technocratisation of society has resulted in increased skill requirements for some and a decrease in skill for others (Hill, 1981; Gordon et al., 1982; King and Martin, 2002; King, 2005; Tignor, 2006). Increased application of technology has in many cases reduced complex mental or physical skills to routine task requirements capable of being performed by most individuals without extensive vocational/technical training. This seems to be as true in the so-called white-collar professions as it is in more typically blue-collar occupations (Johnson, 1982; Moran and Rumble, 2004). Where technology has increased the skill requirements for jobs, this has mainly been true for a small group, namely those who plan the techniques of production.

Furthermore, while some 'high-tech' jobs, such as those of systems analysts, computer programmers, data-processing machine mechanics, and others, are projected to grow between 75% and 149% in the 21st century, their absolute number is small, while increases in unskilled categories as janitors, nurse-aids, fast-food workers and so on will grow at unprecedented rates. Moreover, various economists have in fact concluded that more and more workers will be required by the nature of the economy to take jobs which do not make use of their education and skills, and that formal education certification will be more useful in *getting* rather than in *doing* a job (Levin and Rumberger, 1983; Glewwe, 1999; Hutchful, 2002).

However, there is some evidence that the same trend obtains locally. The Skills and Training Needs Survey notes, for instance, that several companies were losing good and qualified workers because the present occupations under-utilised their skills and levels of training. Furthermore, some specialised companies in non-ferrous metals employ those with limited experience and poor levels of education so that these employees 'would not be able to understand pertinent technological details that would enable them to set up on their own and become a competitive threat' (Ofosuhene, 2000). The Vocational School Tracer Study shows that up to 63% of early leavers and 49% of course completers were doing the same work as colleagues who had not been to the vocational schools but followed the general stream instead. Indeed, it could be argued that the present skills shortage is a socially constructed problem, given that skilled labour is poorly paid and hence will not attract workers, and that there is still occupational segregation in Ghana, which automatically excludes women from vacancies which employers claim they cannot fill (ISSER, 2000).

These caveats serve as an important reminder that employers generally have vested interests when they make claims or register complaints about the educational system. Nevertheless, industry's dissatisfaction with vocational schools does alert us to the fact that schools are notoriously inadequate institutions for vocational training to take place in (Foster, 1965; King and Martin, 2002). The most obvious case which demonstrates the extent to which schools find it difficult to respond to changes in the labour market is the vocational training offered in Ghanaian girls' trade schools. Girls are channelled to work in textile firms. Other skills provided consist of craft-type activities which prepare students for domestic work or the tourist industry. While the focus on industrial sewing might have been functional in the early seventies, when the textile industry was 'the dominant and most important sector of Ghanaian manufacturing establishments and the largest provider of jobs in the private sector' (Ghanaian Times, 15 January 1990), the labour market situation has now changed, without a concomitant reform in vocational schools.

Indeed, due to the availability of cheaper labour in Central and Eastern European countries, general world recession, and changes in government economic policies and in the regulation of exports, the textile industry in Ghana is shrinking drastically, with nine factories closing down over the past five years, with others trimming their work force. In all, 3000 workers have been shed between mid-October 2000 and end-October, 2004 (Daily Graphic, 27 July 2005). But vocational schools continue preparing girls not only for some of the lowest paid, semi-skilled occupations available, but for jobs which might no longer be there.

2. Schools and Industrial Skills for the Future

A second claim of human capital theory is that one can tell which industrial skills will be needed in the future, and that vocational education programmes can therefore engage in the preparation of future manpower needs. Such manpower planning has had an appeal for many governments in the post-war era as they tried to project the types and number of skills needed by the economy in the future so that the educational system would then produce the right number of persons with the appropriate skills. Ghana is no exception, and under the influence of Lewis in the 1950s, successive administrations embarked on a number of manpower planning and forecasting exercises (Tignor, 2006), the latest version being one announced recently by the Ministry of Employment and Training with the intention of conducting comprehensive survey on a national basis to identify labour and skills requirement in order to give 'the government as clear a picture as possible of present and future needs, enabling it to draw up its education and training policies' (Ghanaian Times, 4 June 2000).

Despite the rhetoric accompanying the launching of an exercise which would place Ghana 'in the forefront of future discussion' on the subject in international fora such as the ILO (Daily Graphic, 8 March 1998), the evidence from a number of countries over the past quarter of century has generally discredited attempts at manpower planning and forecasting. Among the reasons that are usually given for the difficulties facing such an exercise are the following (Bulletin of the International Bureau of Education, 1986): the greater frequency and speed of change in the technology/employment area than in the education/training area; the assumption that persons trained in a given occupation will seek that employment; the unreasonable assumption of zero labour substitution; the narrow focus on wage employment in the formal sector to the exclusion of all other forms of economic activity; the focus on growth to the exclusion of equity and social demand; the discrepancies between the actual rates of economic growth and the assumed ones upon which the manpower forecasts are based; the neglect of occupational mobility; and the assumption that particular levels of economic development are reached through specific patterns of educational/occupational structures.

To these we can add Ghana's vulnerability to changes in the international market which play havoc with plans of vocational training initiated in response to projected person-power needs. The mobility of capital makes investment by multinational companies highly unreliable and small states find it particularly difficult to plan ahead (Munbodh, 1987; Elbadawi and Ndulu, 2001; Fosu, 2002; Ndulu et al., 2008). In addition to this, Ghana's recent decision to liberalise its economy has further repercussions on manpower forecasting, given the fact that the only places where the latter has tended to be successful is in centrally planned economies. Here, 'state bureaucracies establish investment policy, set production schedules, organise the distribution of the labour force and determine the content and enrolment level of educational frameworks. Given their strong commitment and actual power to control economic production, it is not surprising that the educational systems of Eastern Europe have been organised to keep in step with, and to be an instrument of, economic development' (Benavot, 1983). In other countries, these attempts have failed (Youdi and Hinchcliffe, 1985; Middleton et al, 1993; Yang, 1998; World Bank, 2003; Ndulu et al., 2008), often miserably, and have in fact generated unemployment because 'the skills assessed as of today that would be needed twenty years from now, will be very different from those that the economy will be actually demanding in the future' (Psacharopoulos, 1991).

3. Vocational Education and Career Paths

In fact, most research carried out in developing and developed countries, shows that the assumption that students will find, or even look for work in the area related to their training is unfounded. Lewis and Lewis (1985) review research reporting trends in the Caribbean, for instance, and tracer studies carried out in a number of islands in the late seventies and early eighties confirm general findings elsewhere that large percentages – between 25% and 33% -

of vocational students were not working in the course-related jobs. Similar results have been obtained from tracer studies with students following vocational tracks in American high schools. In this case, only 27.4% of the employed graduates had a training-related job 1 to 10 years after leaving high school (Bishop, 1986). Another study showed that only 21% of employed vocational graduates had a training-related job two years after finishing high school (Campbell et al., 1986). The countries which have reported higher percentages of graduates in training-related jobs have been those which like Germany, have employers who are heavily involved in the training offered to students.

A number of studies carried out in Ghana evince many of the problems outlined above with reference to both job orientation and job placement. The 2000 data from the Vocational Secondary School Research Project Questionnaire (VSSRPQ) suggests that in intention at least, 61.3% of male students and 57.8% of female students think their main job will be in the vocational area they have studied at school. Only 9.1% of male students said they would be working in an unrelated area. The percentage for females in this case was significantly higher, with 22.4% saying they would be working in a different field altogether. It is also significant to point out that 20.3% of the female and 29.6% of the male students did not answer this question, suggesting a degree of uncertainty about their occupational futures, and that young adults entering the skilled and semi-skilled labour market segments are more prone to take up what is available than to choose jobs. In other words, there are jobs looking for people, rather than people looking for jobs (Roberts, 1977; Moran and Rumble, 2004). This readiness to enter the labour market when openings presented themselves can be partly understood when 47.6% of the female and 47.7% of the male students said they were not quite sure whether it would be easy or difficult to find employment on leaving school, while 23.1% of the girls and 11.7% of the boys declared it would be difficult to find a job.

The best way to find out which occupations vocational students have in fact taken up is through tracer studies. One such study was carried out by the Guidance and Counselling Services (2001) of the Ministry of Education in September and October 2001 with all June 2001 school-leavers. This shows that of the 350 male vocational graduates who replied, representing 82.5% of the total who received the questionnaire, 20.9% were in manufacturing work, 7.3% reported that they were working in the tourist industry, while another 13.2% said they were working in the service sector. The last two figures show that 20.5% of all vocational school-leavers were in an occupation which trade schools had not prepared them for. In addition to this, one cannot assume that those in manufacturing work were doing training-related tasks. This is borne out not only by other tracer studies reported below, but also by data obtained from interviews with vocational secondary school heads who noted that students applied to fill dockyard vacancies, for instance, irrespective of the trade they were taking at school. Data for girls indicated that 72.1% of those who replied were in manufacturing work, and, given employment opportunities for women in Ghana, were almost certainly in textile factories, 4.8% were in tourism, 2.9% in services, while a full 15.1% remained 'at home'. In any case, 89% of the girls said they would not remain in full-time employment once they had children.

Tracer studies were carried out by the present author. This tracer study (henceforth referred to as TSTS) set out to contact two groups of students, early school-leavers and course completers, who entered employment in 2001/2002. In the case of early school-leavers, 71.6% were working in jobs totally unrelated to the trade they had studied at school. The course-completers were more likely to have benefited from their trade training, since 'only'

38.7% had found employment in course-unrelated occupations. This could mean that students take some time until they actually find a job related to their training.

4. Rates-of-Return for Vocational Students

If a key dimension in the evaluation of educational programmes is the benefits they provide to their clients – students – then it becomes important to explore at some length whether vocational schooling gives students any advantages in the labour market when compared to 'non-vocational' students. In other words, it is not sufficient to evaluate the rates-of-return of vocational schooling for the nation, but also for its graduates. Most studies which have attempted to address this issue have also attempted to answer one or more of the following questions:

- Do vocational students find employment quickly?
- Are they more likely to be unemployed?
- How do their wages compare with those received by non-vocational students?
- What conditions of work do they enjoy?

An extensive empirical literature has developed over the last 35 years, comparing the labour market outcomes (in terms of earnings and employment) of vocational school leavers with those from lower cost general schooling, mainly at the secondary level. Most studies displayed low rates of return on societal investment in vocational education (compared with those from general, academic schooling). Comparatively low returns on vocational schooling have been reported in many studies, particularly for low-income countries, where vocational education capacity exceeds labour market demand and the external efficiency of SVTE is low. Examples include Benin (Rasara, 1988), Mozambique (Ziderman, 1997), Niger (Mingat et al, 1989) and Somalia (Chapman and Windham, 1985). However, other studies find that graduates of general and vocational schools earn about the same but the higher costs of vocational schools result in higher rates of return to general, academic schooling. Two such studies are set in the Cote d'Ivoire (Grootaert, 1990) and in Indonesia (Clark, 1983); nevertheless, consistent results are reported for Peru (Bellew and Moock, 1990).

Consequently, the main thrust of these empirical studies has been to argue against vocational schooling on cost-benefit grounds: the attack has been led by George Psacharopoulos and his associates at the World Bank. A number of research studies have qualified this established orthodoxy, reporting rather more favourable outcomes for SVTE. And a series of studies for the USA (reviewed by Bishop, 1989) focused more closely than earlier studies on the type of jobs held by vocational school leavers and on the relationship between the vocational course specialty studied and subsequent employment. However, in contrast with the earlier work, these concluded that vocational education can confer labour market advantages in terms of participation, employment and wages for those high school leavers who work in jobs related to the vocational courses followed at school, while vocational school leavers working outside their training specialty fare rather no better than workers who undertook general academic streams. Also consistent results are reported for Israel (Neuman and Ziderman, 1991), Brazil (Arriagada and Ziderman, 1992), China (Min and Tsang, 1990), Switzerland (Sager, 2008), and for Hong Kong (Chung, 1990). In any case, a central factor in these studies has been the availability of employment opportunities and the match between vocational skills and available jobs.

With regard to availability of employment for vocational students, the evidence reported by a number of countries is mixed and therefore inconclusive. Some claim that students trained in a vocation do better in getting jobs than students opting for a general education (Freedland and Little, 1980; Arriagada and Ziderman, 1992; Aypay, 2003; Chappell, 2003; Hawley, 2003; Hall and Raffo, 2004; King, 2005). A study carried out with 12,000 young people by the U.S. National Centre for Research and Vocational Education, for example, found that the more vocational courses the student takes, the more likely s/he is to find a job (Campbell, 1981). Depending on the condition and performance of the labour market, Norwegian vocational students do in fact do better in terms of earning, feeling of autonomy on the job, participation in trade unions, and other such measures. These advantages are especially significant when we consider that vocational track students have often stayed for a shorter period in schools (Lindbekk, 1989). However, a review of income returns to graduates from academic and vocational secondary education in several Asian and African countries suggests that for many countries, there are short-term returns for vocational education graduates, but in the long-term, the pattern changed to the benefit of those from academic lines (Hawley, 2003; King, 2005). In France, graduates in the general education schools come off better in the short-term as well (McMahon, 1988).

Research has also indicated that for those who do not pursue their studies at college/post-secondary level, the high school curriculum had little effect on labour market outcomes, irrespective of whether that curriculum was general or vocational (Myer and Wise, 1983; King, 2005; Sager, 2008). A major study by the Bureau of Labour Statistics concluded that of the 53 million Americans employed in jobs which required training, only 5% received it in high school vocational classes. The same study also indicates that business/office studies, often followed by female students, represent one of the few vocational areas that do give an advantage in the labour market (Carey and Eck, 1984). Psacharopoulos (1987) concludes that there is really no hard evidence that returns for individuals, or for society generally, are any better with vocational streams, even when one looks at their effect in developing countries. Indeed, vocational education students are more likely to spend longer periods unemployed. Tilak (1987) arrives at much the same conclusions after reviewing fourteen studies carried out in developing countries.

Given the nature of the conflicting evidence available, some have argued that it would be safe to conclude that training in certain occupational areas gives more benefits to students than others (Mertens, 1983; Arriagada and Ziderman, 1992; Ziderman, 1997; Aypay, 2003; Chappell, 2003; Hall and Raffo, 2004; Moran and Rumble, 2004; Vlaardingerbroek et al, 2007), and that vocational education can make a small positive difference for some of the people some of the time (Claus, 1990; Hawley, 2003; World Bank, 2003; Tignor, 2006).

There are a number of problems which must be highlighted before the Ghanaian empirical data are compared with that obtaining from international studies. A key issue which is not often raised is that an important variable in the rates of return for students might not be whether s/he followed a vocational or general track, but the nature of the reward structure of the labour market which absorbs school-leavers (Lewis and Lewis, 1985; Elbadawi, and Ndulu, 2001; Hawley, 2003; Vlaardingerbroek et al, 2007). A second problem is that when comparison is made between the rates of return for vocational and for general students, it is often forgotten that these two types of tracks attract different 'types' of students, with the vocational catering for what are often socio-economically depressed groups of students. Even if these achieve less, in financial terms than general education students, one would have to see whether their rates of return would have been as good or bad had they too joined the general stream (Moura Castro, 1987; Lewin, 1993; Bennell, 1995; Chappell, 2003; Hawley, 2003).

A related issue is that vocational students are a 'self-selected group' likely to possess not only similar backgrounds, but also skills and aspirations which are different from those of the groups with which they are compared. Thus, 'differences which appear between vocational and non-vocational groups at the completion of a programme may reflect not programme impact, but prior differences which escaped detection of the survey measures. Alternatively, such differences may reflect differential interactions between certain kinds of students and certain programme features' (Claus, 1990). Furthermore, differences between the results obtained by male and female students reflect the different opportunities and rewards that a segmented labour market presents to the different genders.

In addition, most of rates-of-return studies do not explain why vocational education graduates tend to do less well. The reason for this may be in the different value that specific skills as against general skills have for employers. The former are those that are useful to one employer, while the latter are those which every employer finds productive. The employer need not pay narrowly skilled workers higher wages than those prevailing for unskilled labourers, since the specific skills are useless to any other firm and there is no incentive for other employers to bid specifically skilled workers away. However, in the case of general skills, employers will try to poach workers by offering them higher wages. Thus, while it behoves employers to train specific skills, the general skilled persons are more productive to all firms, and their wages must be increased in order to hire them. With specific skills, the benefits of that training may be captured by firms instead of workers (Grubb, 1978; Lauglo, 1992; Ziderman, 1997; Dehmel, 2005).

The Vocational School Tracer Studies carried out in Ghana indicate that vocational students do not generally encounter many difficulties in finding a niche in the local labour market, though obviously one needs to examine the status of that niche, preferably in comparison with the sorts of opportunities available to students who graduate from other schools. Over 80% of early leavers and 93.8% of course completers who responded to the TSTS questionnaires were in employment, with most 60% of the former and 87% of the latter finding a job within six months of leaving school. With a situation of almost full employment, this is not surprising and the relative advantage or disadvantage of vocational school students is not clear. However, an analysis of the 16-18 year old young adults registering for unemployment showed that the most at risk were, first, those who had only primary schooling, and then those who had attended vocational schools. 31.7% (n=150) were male students who had completed the trade school course, while 27.9% (n=135) had left vocational schools early. Females were not highly represented in the list of registered unemployed (ISSER, 2000).

In addition to this, the TSTS shows that most vocational school students found themselves in unskilled (46% of early leavers; 8.9% of course completers) and semi-skilled work (40.5% and 41.5% respectively). The Skills and Training Needs Survey confirms this pattern, noting that 11% of the workers from a technical education level were found to be employed in unskilled occupations, and considers this to be a 'disturbing result' which called for further investigation (Ofosuhene, 2000). Almost 70% of early leavers and 45% of course completers felt that somebody who had never attended a trade school could have performed the same type of work they were presently doing.

The computation of the financial rates-of-return for vocational track students compared with general track students is complex in itself because, as noted earlier, there are a number of variables involved, so that any final conclusions might be referring to elements other than programme effects. A major factor to be considered is the reward structure in Ghana, where almost twenty years of PNDC/NDC administration reduced wage differentials between manual and non-manual labour as well as between different working grades (Daily Graphic, 9 December, 2000). As Carnoy (1990) has pointed out with reference to societies which embarked on a socialist programme, 'The individual material cost of not doing well in school is greatly reduced, and so is the material payoff of reaching higher levels of schooling. The motivation for high achievement in school comes in part from the continued (but smaller) differences in income, but more from nonmaterial rewards (such as easier, more prestigious jobs and political power) and from pressures of social responsibility (a more productive life and a greater contribution to the people-nation)'.

The particularity of the reward structure of the Ghanaian labour market is perceived by students, and is reflected in their beliefs about the effectiveness of schooling in increasing earning power. The perceptions were once more influenced by the gender of respondents. Data from the VSSRPQ show that 27.8% of boys in Vocational Schools said they were sure that vocational schooling led to jobs which were as well paid as jobs which required academic schooling. A further 38.1% stated they were not sure about what was most remunerative, while 31.9% indicated that academic schooling gave better rates of return. However, girls seemed to think that vocational schooling was generally less remunerative, with 47.2% expecting their counterparts in general schools to earn more money than themselves. 36.1% were not quite sure, while only 7.9% thought that vocational schooling put them ahead, in terms of earning power, than others.

While vocational school students were generally uncertain as to whether vocational schooling gave them more earning power than general schooling, the VSSRPQ data show that they expected their training to contribute to higher earnings in the future, when this was compared to the earnings of untrained workers in similar work environments. This was true of 83.1% of male students and 71.9% of females. Indeed 51% of the former, but only 15.7% of the latter thought it would pay to invest in further vocational education. The tracer studies suggest that this faith in schooling decreases, but is still significantly high when male vocational school graduates look back from the vantage point of employment to comment on whether further study in a trade would have given them better job possibilities. Thus, the TSTS with early leavers shows that 64% thought that had they stayed longer in a vocational school, they would have had better job possibilities, while 46.7% of the course completers were of the same opinion. However, a significantly high percentage from both groups 31.9% and 37.7% respectively, felt that further study would not have made much of a difference in job opportunities and rewards.

If one compares the above expectations with actual wages earned by 2000/2001 vocational school graduates represented in the TSTS, it then becomes clear that a full 45% of early school leavers were not succeeding in earning the minimum wage (Guidance and Counselling Services, 2001). As to course completers (King and Martin, 2002), these were earning, in general, slightly above the minimum wage. It is significant that 43.1% of early school leavers and 42.4% of course completers remarked that low pay was a major drawback at their place of work. This does not represent the whole picture. If one is to put a value on the vocational training that vocational school students receive, one has to keep in mind the phenomenon of Ghana's underground economy, which accounts for between 10 and 15% of the GNP (Glewwe, 1999). From the VSSRPQ data and interviews with vocational secondary school students it became clear that the latter were likely utilising their vocational skills in a second, unofficial job. Thus, 36% of the male and 6.1% of the female students who answered the VSSRPQ expressed their intention to have a second job. By far the greater majority of male vocational school students aspired to work with governmental or parastatal bodies.

The Skills and Training Needs Survey reported similar data, with 42% making the Government sector their first choice (Ofosuhene, 2000). The TSTS shows that, by and large, these intentions seem to be followed when students enter the labour market, with, on average, 25% being employed by the state and 45% by private industry. While a very small number, five students in all, had in fact set up on their own, it is likely that many of them were earning over and above their wage by doing other jobs. The Skills and Training Needs Survey notes that many vocational school students aspired for government jobs because of the job security that sector offered, and also because it left them enough time to work part-time elsewhere. Informal, unstructured interviews with vocational school students revealed that some preferred to first work with the government until they had learned their trade well, and once they had obtained experience and expertise, they intended to leave state employment and start their own enterprise, perhaps by turning a secondary job into a primary one. Apparently, no information is available as to whether these secondary jobs correspond to skills learnt at school. If this were found out to be so, then vocational schooling might be contributing not to development in the formal but the underground economy.

CONCLUSION

With regard to Foster's theme, relating to the appropriate location of skills training to meet the needs of industry, skills preparation in vocational schools is usually less cost-effective than employer-based training. The cost-effectiveness of employer training stems from lower training costs, the use of more up-to-date machinery and the ready match that may be made between skills demanded and training supplied, each within the context of the enterprise. Enterprise-based training may take the contrasting forms of informal learning, formal structured training on-the-job or regulated apprenticeship; yet by definition, it is demand driven and thus oriented to the needs of the market (Ziderman, 2003). However, in low-income countries, where the modern sector is undeveloped, size of enterprise small, managerial competencies limited, and trade associations poorly developed, then the enterprise base may not have the capacity to provide adequate training to meet industry's needs, particularly structured training at low cost. Since the publication of Foster's famous article, the appropriate role to be accorded to SVTE, both within the schooling and the training systems, has been an issue of intense debate.

Secondary Vocational/Technical Education (SVTE) is concerned with pre-employment skills preparation; yet this concept is increasingly coming under challenge by the changing needs of labour markets. The ongoing pace of industrial restructuring, product innovation and new technologies are changing the nature of the work environment (World Bank, 2003). In my opinion, companies will require in their workers attributes of adaptability and trainability rather than the possession of a fixed toolkit of skills. SVTE will need to become less specifically geared towards providing the skills necessary for a particular job. It will need to offer a broader training, emphasizing the need for subsequent worker learning, trainability and flexibility. In this sense SVTE will move closer in concept and practice to academic secondary schools and at the same time closer towards the world of employment.

Clearly, this paper has shown that the economic goals established for vocational/technical secondary schools have not, in fact, been reached, since these schools are not responding – and cannot respond – adequately enough to the economic needs of the nation, and are most probably not bringing enough returns to the students who follow courses there. Large numbers of vocational students take up main jobs unrelated to their training while most female vocational school students are more likely to quit their job as soon as they have had children. As a result, the nation cannot recoup investment made in its attempt to develop a skilled workforce. All these reasons militate against vocational schools performing the direct economic function that was intended for them. The most that one can claim is that these schools fulfil an *indirect* economic function:

- By building up a technological culture in the labour force (though it seems that high rates of absenteeism, as well as outdated technology in schools, jeopardise this function), and
- By directing a percentage of students away from academic education and into blue collar occupational paths.

The second goal could never be a declared intention for schools in a nation which overtly claims that justice and democracy are its guiding values.

Apparently, vocational schooling does not seem to bring much in the way of advantages to students who are channelled, or choose to go to that particular educational structure. Vocational students are more likely to be unemployed than students from other types of schools, and generally find work as unskilled and semi-skilled workers, so that they are ultimately engaged in doing work which others who have not gone to vocational schools can do. In addition, they are exposed to a restricted general curriculum which should be considered a disadvantage, not only from the civic but also from the industrial point of view.

Lastly, an evaluation of the returns of vocational schooling for the nation and for the individual student must be placed within a macro social-economic context. Whether this kind of schooling will bring more or less advantages or disadvantages will depend on such factors as the rate of growth of the overall economy, and particularly of the sector which will make use of the vocational skills taught; the structure of incentives and disincentives that influence the allocation of available specialised labour; the quality and relevance of the education that vocational students bring with them to the labour market, and so on and so forth. Government policies, such as in increasing or decreasing wage differentials between blue and white-collar work, will also have a direct impact on the attractiveness of, and/or rates-of-return for, vocational schooling. In other words, the reasons for the economic success or failure of vocational schools need to be identified not only from within the educational institution, but also from the outside. Also other variables, that have nothing to do with education as such, must be carefully examined.

REFERENCES

Al-Samarrai, S., Reilly, B. (2005) Education, employment and earnings of secondary school leavers in Tanzania: evidence from a tracer study PRUS Working Paper No 31

Antwi, M. K. (1992) *Education, Society and Development in Ghana*, Accra: Unimax Publishers

Arriagada, A. M. and Ziderman, A. (1992) *Vocational Secondary Schooling, Occupational Choice, and Earnings in Brazil*, World Bank Policy Research Working Papers WPS 1037, The World Bank, Washington DC

Aypay, A. (2003) The tough choice at high school door: an investigation of factors that lead to general or vocational schools, *International Journal of Educational Development* 23(5), 517-527

Bellew, R. and Moock, P (1990) Vocational and technical education in Peru *Economics of Education Review* 9: 365-376

Ben-abdallah, M. (1986) *Statement on the State of the Educational System by the PNDC Secretary for Education and Culture*, Ministry of Education, Accra

Benavot, A. (1983) The rise and decline of vocational schooling, *Sociology of Education* 56, 63-76

Bennell, P. (1995) *General versus Vocational Secondary Education in Developing Countries: A Review of Rates of Evidence* Brighton, UK University of Sussex Institute of Development Studies

Berg, I. (1970) *Education and Jobs: The Great Training Robbery*, Praeger, New York

Bishop, J. (1986) Occupationally specific training in High Schools In *Re-Visioning Vocational Education in the Secondary School* (edited by Copa, G. H., Plihal, , J. and Johnson, M. A.) Minnesota Research and Development Centre for Vocational Education, Minnesota

Bishop, J (1989) Occupational training in high school: when does it pay off? *Economics of Education Review* 8: 1-15

Blackmore, J. (1990) The test and context of vocationalism, *Journal of Curriculum Studies* 22 (2), 177-184

Blaug, M. (1973) *Education and the Employment Problem in Developing Countries* ILO, Geneva

Blaug, M. (1970) *An Introduction to the Economics of Education* Harmondsworth: Penguin

Bowles, S. (1973) Understanding unequal economic opportunity *American Economic Review* 63, 14-23

Bowman, J. (1988) Links between general and vocational education: does the one enhance the other? *International Review of Education* 34 (2), 149-171

Braverman, H. (1974) *Labour and Monopoly Capital Monthly Review Press* New York.

Bulletin of the International Bureau of Education (1986) *Special Issue on education and employment*, No. 238/9, Unesco, Paris

Campbell, P. (1981) *Employment Experiences of Students with Varying Participation in Vocational Education, National Centre for Research in Vocational Education*, Ohio State University, Columbus

Campbell, P. B., Bassinger, K. S., Dauner, M. B. and Parkes, M. A. (1986) *Outcomes of Vocational Education for Women, Minorities, the Handicapped and the Poor*, The National Centre for Research in Vocational Education, Ohio State University, Columbus

Carey, M. and Eck, A. (1984) How workers get their training, *Occupational Outlook Quarterly* 28 (4), 22-28

Carnoy, M. (1990) Education and the Transition State In *Education and Social Transition in the Third World* (edited by Carnoy, M. and Samoff, J.) Princeton University Press, Princeton

Chapman, D. W. and Windham, D. M. (1985) Academic program 'failures' and the vocational school fallacy: policy issues in secondary education in Somalia *International Journal of Educational Development* 5: 269-281

Chappell, C. (2003) Researching vocational education and training: where to from here? *Journal of Vocational Education and Training*, 55(1), 21-32

Chung, Y-P. (1990) Educated-misemployment in Hong Kong: earnings effects of employment in unmatched fields of work, *Economics of Education Review* 9: 343-350

Clark, D. (1983) *How Secondary School Graduates Perform in the Labour Market: a study of Indonesia* World Bank Working Paper No. 615 Washington The World Bank

Claus, J. (1990) Opportunity or inequality in vocational education?: a qualitative investigation. *Curriculum Inquiry* 29 (1) 7-39

Collins, R. (1979) *The Credential Society*. Academic Press, New York

Daehlen, M. (2005) Changes in job values during education *Journal of Education and Work* 18 (4) 385-400

Daily Graphic (1986) Junior secondary school (JSS) reform 6 November: 1-2, *Daily Graphic* Accra

Daily Graphic (1998) The Minister of Works and Employment 8 March: 2-3, *Daily Graphic* Accra

Daily Graphic (2000) Wage differentials between manual and non-manual labour 9 December: 3-4, *Daily Graphic* Accra

Daily Graphic (2002) The need for vocational secondary school training, 9 September: 2-3 *Daily Graphic* Accra

Daily Graphic (2005) 5,000 Job loses in textile, poultry and rice industry, 27 July: 1-2, *Daily Graphic* Accra

Dehmel, A. (2005) *The Role of Vocational Education and Training in Promoting Lifelong Learning in Germany and England*, Symposium Books, Oxford

Elbadawi, I. A. and Ndulu, B. J. (2001) *Economic Development in Sub-Saharan Africa: Proceedings of the Eleventh World Congress of the International Economic Association*, Tunis

Emerson, R. M., Fretz, R. and Shaw, L. L. (1996) *Writing ethnographic notes*, Chicago, University of Chicago Press

Fiah, S. (1981) *An examination of the role of education in supporting the rural economy of Southern Ghana*, Unpublished Doctoral Thesis: University of Hull

Foster, P. J. (1965) The vocational school fallacy in development planning. In C. A. Anderson and M. Bowman (eds.) *Education and Economic Development*, Aldine, Chicago

Fosu, A. (2002) International trade and labour market adjustment in developing countries in Greenaway, D., Upward, R. and Wakelin, K. (eds.) *Trade, Investment, Migration and Labour Market Adjustment*, Palgrave Macmillan, London

Freeland, J. E. and Little, R. D. (1980) Long-term returns to vocational training, *Journal of Human Resources* 85, 19-27

Ghanaian Times (1990) The rise and fall of the textile industry, 15 January: 1-2 *Ghanaian Times* Accra

Ghanaian Times (1999) Vocational training in secondary schools: 5 April: 3-4 *Ghanaian Times*, Accra

Ghanaian Times (2000) Labour and skills requirements: 4 June: 2-3 *Ghanaian Times*, Accra

Glaser, B. G. and Strauss, A. L. (1967) *The Discovery of Grounded Theory: Strategies for Qualitative Research.* Aldine, Chicago

Glewwe, P. (1999) *The Economics of School Quality Investment in Developing Countries: An Empirical Study of Ghana*, Centre for The Study of African Economics, University of Oxford

Gordon, D., Edwards, R. and Reich, M. (1982) *Segmented Work, Divided Workers: Historical Transformation of Labour in the United States*, Cambridge University Press, Cambridge

Grootaert, C. (1990) Returns to formal and informal vocational education in Cote d'Ivoire: the role of the structure of the labour market *Economics of Education Review* 9: 309-320

Grubb, W. N. (1978) The phoenix of vocationalism: hope deferred is hope denied. *New Directions for Education and Work*, Spring 71-89

Grubb, W. N. (1985) The convergence of educational systems and the role of vocationalism *Comparative Education Review* 29, 526-548

Guidance and Counselling Services (2001) Results of a Tracer Study held in September/October, 2001, Ministry of Education, Accra, mimeo

Hall, D. and Raffo, C. (2004) Re-engaging 14-16 year-olds with their schooling through work-related learning *Journal of Vocational Education and Training* 56 (1), 69-79

Hawley, J. D. (2003) Comparing the payoff to vocational and academic credentials in Thailand over time *International Journal of Educational Development* 23, 607-625

Hill, S. (1981) *Competition and Control at Work*, Heinemann, London

Honny, L. A. (1999) Reshaping vocational training: hopeful signs from a Ghanaian experience, in K. King and S. McGrath (eds.) *Enterprise in Africa: Between Poverty and Growth*, Intermediate Technology Publications, Southampton

Hutchful, E. (2002) *Ghana's Adjustment Experience: The Paradox of Reform*, James Currey, Oxford

ISSER (2000) Ghana Statistics, *Institute of Scientific, Social and Economic Research (ISSER)* Accra

Jencks, C. (1972) *Inequality: A Reassessment.* Basic, New York

Johnson, D. (ed.) (1982) Class and Social Development: A New Theory of the Middle Class. Sage, Beverly Hills

King, K. (2005) Re-targeting schools, skills and jobs in Kenya: quantity, quality and outcomes *International Journal of Educational Development* 25(4), 423-435

King, K. (1990) *Training and Structural Adjustment: Images from Ghana and Nigeria and the Impact of Structural Adjustment on Technical and Vocational Education and Training Systems*, Occasional Paper No 29

King, K. and Martin, C. (2002) The Vocational school fallacy revisited: education, aspiration and work in Ghana 1959-2000 *International Journal of Educational Development* 22 5-26

King, K. and McGrath, S. (2002) *Globalisation, Enterprise and Knowledge: Education, Training and Development in Africa*, Monographs in International Education, Symposium Books, Wallingford

Lauglo, J. (1987) Practical subjects in Kenyan academic secondary schools In: *Vocationalising Education* (edited by Lauglo, J. and Lillis, K.) Pergamon Press, Oxford

Lauglo, J. (1992) *Vocational Training: Analysis of Policy and Modes*, International Institute for Educational Planning, Paris

Levin, H. M. and Rumberger, R. W. (1983) *The Educational Implications of High Technology*, Institute for Research on Educational Finance and Government, Stanford, Ca.

Lewin, K. (1993) Investing in technical and vocational education: a review of evidence *The Vocational Aspect of Education* 45 (3): 217-227

Lewis, T. and Lewis, M. V. (1985) Vocational education in the commonwealth Caribbean and the United States *Comparative Education* 21 (2), 157-171

Lewis, W. A. (1953) *Gold Coast and Industrialisation: A Report*, Government Printing Press, Accra

Lindbekk, T. (1989) Education for life: vocational education and social integration in Norway, *Comparative Education* 25 (1), 19-28

Mandebele, C. and Ephraim, D. (2008) High school vocational programmes: self-reported perceptions of vocational teachers in Swaziland *Journal of Vocational Education and Training* 60 (3): 315-325

Mcmahon, W. W. (1988) The economics of vocational and technical education: do the benefits outweigh the costs? *International Review of Education* 34, 38-54

Mertens, D. (1983) The vocational graduate in the labour market, *Phi Delta Kappan* 64 (5), 360-362

Middleton, J., Adams, A. V. and Ziderman, A. (1993) *Skills for Productivity: Vocational Education and Training in Developing Countries* University Press New York: Oxford

Min, W. and Tsang, M. C. (1990) Vocational education and productivity: a case study of the Beijing General Auto industry Compnay *Economics of Education* Review 9: 351-364

Mingat, A., Jarousse, J-P. and Richard, M. (1989) *L'Enseignement Technique Court au Niger Une evaluation par le marche*. Dijon: IREDU

Ministry of Information (1986) *Tertiary Education: Proposed Reforms*, Government Printing Press, Accra

Moran, L. and Rumble, G. (2004) *Vocational Education and Training through Open and Distance Learning*, Routledge Falmer, London and New York

Moura Castro, C. DE (1987) Is vocational education really that bad? *International Labour Review* 126 (5), 603-610

Myer, R. H. and Wise, D. A. (1983) High school preparation and early labour market experience. In *Youth Joblessness and Unemployment* (edited by Freeman, R. B. and Medoff, J. L.), University of Chicago Press, Chicago

Ndulu, B. J., O'Connell, S. A., Bates, R. H., Collier, P. and Soludo, C. C. (2008) *The Political Economy of Growth in Africa, 1960-2000* Cambridge University Press

Neuman, S. and Ziderman, A. (1991) Vocational schooling, occupational matching, and labour market earnings in Israel *Journal of Human Resources* 21: 256-281

Nye, B. and Hedges, L. (2001) The influence of elementary school class size on ninth grade math test scores, *Journal of International Education* 69, 218-233

Oakes, J. (1986) Beyond tinkering: reconstructing vocational education. In Copa, G. H. et al., op. cit.

Ofosuhene, K. (2000) *Review of Skills Survey To-Date* Mimeo, Accra

Osei, G. M. (2001) *An Examination of Policy and Practice in Ghanaian Education, with Special Reference to the Junior Secondary School Reform*, Doctoral Thesis, University of Oxford, Oxford

Osei, G. M. (2003) Issues arising from an examination of the junior secondary school reform of 1987 in Ghana, *Educational Studies* 29 (2/3), 141-177

Osei, G. M. (2004) The 1987 junior secondary school reform in Ghana: vocational or pre-vocational in nature? *International Review of Education* 50 (5-6), 425-446

Osei, G. M. (2006) Teachers in Ghana: issues of training, remuneration and effectiveness, *International Journal of Educational Development* 26, 38-51

Osei, G. M. (2009) *Curriculum Innovation and its problems: The Case of Ghana's Junior Secondary Schools*, New York: Nova Science Publishers

Osei, G. M. (2007) Vocationalising secondary education: the junior secondary schooling reform of 1987 in Ghana, *Educational Review* 59 (1): 71-85

Oxenham, J. (1987) What do employers want from education? In: Lauglo, J. and Lillis, K., op. cit.

Psacharopoulos, G. (1987) To vocationalise or not to vocationalise: that is the curriculum question. *International Review of Education* 33 (2), 187-211

Psacharopoulos, G. (1988) Editorial introduction *International Review of Education* 34 (2), 143-148

Psacharopoulos, G. (1991) Education and work: the perennial mismatch and ways to solve it. *The Vocational Aspect of Education* 114, 18-27

Rasara, J. B. (1988) *Les Enseingement Moyens General et Technique au Benin: devinir des diplomes coutes de rendement internes des etudes*. Dejon: IREDU

Roberts, K. (1977) The social conditions, consequences and limitations of careers guidance, *British Journal of Guidance and Counselling* 5 (1), 1-9

Sager, F. (2008) Securing the long-term bases of the dual system: a realistic evaluation of apprenticeship marketing in Switzerland *Journal of Vocational Education* 60 (3): 327-341

Semple, N. M. (1987) Vocational education: missing link *Peabody Journal of Education* 26 (2), 70-90

Small, R. (2005) *Marx and Education* Ashgate Publishing Ltd, Aldershot

Sobel, I. (1978) The human capital revolution in economic development: its current history and status. *Comparative Education Review* 22, 27-34

Tignor, R. L. (2005) *W. Arthur Lewis and The Birth of Development Economics* Princeton University Press Princeton NJ; London

Tilak, J. B. (1987) Economics of Vocationalisation: a review of evidence, *Canadian and International Education* 17, 45-62

Tilak, J. B. G. (1988) Vocational education in South Asia: problems and prospects. *International Review of Education* 34 (2), 244-257

Violas, P. C. (1981) Reflections on theories of human capital, skills training and vocational education *Educational Theory* 31 (2), 137-151

Vlaardingerbroek, B., Dallal, K., Rizkallah, G. and Rabah, J. (2007) A tracer study of Lebanese upper secondary school students *International Journal of Educational Development* 27 564-571

Vlaardingerbroek, B. (2001) Botswana secondary students' perceptions of the education/employment nexus *International Journal of Educational Development* 21 (3): 315-329

World Bank (2003) *Skills for Productivity: Vocational Education and Training in Developing Countries*, Oxford University Press, New York

Yang, Jin (1998) General or vocational? tough choice in the Chinese education policy *International Journal of Educational Development* 8 (4): 289-304

Youdi, R. B. and Hinchcliffe, K. (1985) *Forecasting Skilled Manpower Needs: The Experience of Eleven Countries*, Unesco, IIEP, Paris

Ziderman, A. (1997) National programmes in technical and vocational education: economic and educational relationships *Journal of Vocational Education and Training* 49 (3), 351-366

Ziderman, A. (2003) *Financing Vocational Training to meet Policy Objectives: Sub-Saharan Africa*, African Region Human Development Series, Washington DC

In: New Research in Education Adult, Medical and Vocational ISBN 978-1-60741-873-3
Editors: Edmondo Balistrieri and Giustino DeNino © 2009 Nova Science Publishers, Inc.

Chapter 5

USING ICT RESOURCES IN PROJECT-BASED LEARNING WITHIN A VOCATIONAL EDUCATION AND TRAINING ENVIRONMENT

Helen Bound and Annette Salter
Univrsity of Tasmania, Tasmania, Australia

ABSTRACT

There is a demand for more flexible delivery approaches in Vocational Education and Training, which has led to greater exploration of the use of Information and Communications Technology (ICT). This chapter describes a collaborative approach used by a small team of trade teachers seeking to develop ICT resources to help meet the requirements of their Registered Training Organization (RTO). The institutional policy of the RTO is shifting to favor a constructivist, project-based, approach to learning over traditional instructional pedagogy, as well as industry and individual requirements for more flexible learning options.

Key words: instruction, ICT resources, project-based learning

INTRODUCTION

This chapter includes a report on research that was supported by a grant from SIMERR. Tasmania. This group is part of the National Centre of Science, Information, and Communication Technology, and Mathematics Education for Rural and Regional Australia. SIMERR is based at the University of New England in Armidale, New South Wales, Australia. This chapter traces the progress of a small team of trade teachers in a public Registered Training Organization (RTO) seeking to address the current issues of their flexible delivery program. They have taken a distinctive approach, which aims to enhance flexible delivery while maintaining and improving the quality of learning. The project involves the teaching team working in conjunction with the RTO's flexible delivery management team and two researchers (the authors). The team (a small group working within a large team of trade teachers) recognizes the need for the teachers to be active participants in many aspects of the change process, to provide opportunities for the teachers to develop their thinking about learning styles and approaches, and for the teachers to have greater control over the ICT resources and materials embedded in the program. Towards these ends a community of learners approach has been adopted, in which the team of teachers, the flexible delivery management team, and the researchers collaborate in the development of the new flexible curriculum. The teachers will be the key drivers when designing, producing, and implementing the learning technology materials.

The introduction of ICT resources is often considered to be the solution to the demand for flexible delivery. However, the problem is to find pedagogical models that allow the introduction of technologies to the learning process in ways that enhance rather than reduce the quality of the learning activities.

BACKGROUND

Although there is a growing body of work on the use of ICT resources in school and university settings, there is limited knowledge of how these tools influence teaching and learning practices in Vocational Education and Training (Kilpatrick and Bound, 2003), particularly in the teaching of trades. In an institutional and policy environment which has historically supported the use of an instructional pedagogy, the question is how to change and develop teaching practices. The Australian Flexible Learning Framework for the National Vocational Education and Training system notes that:

> The overarching policy task for all VET stakeholders is … to encourage the use of the internet and information technologies … to meet the needs of learners. … [T]here is an even more important driver – the needs of individual and industry clients for more flexible learning options (ANTA, 2001, p. 6).

Flexible learning places the onus on the provider to meet the needs of industry and individual learners. Flexible learning requires a change from delivering learning in fixed 2-week blocks of time for apprentices released from industry to delivering learning at the workplace, at home and at the learning institution within flexible timeframes. It also endorses "a change to the mindset of teachers and learners" (ANTA, 1998, p. 4) where the teacher "is no longer central to the passing on of information but to the resourcing of the learners, who will then research and absorb the information" (ibid.). The RTO and team involved in this project were highly cognizant of these policy directions and are actively seeking ways of meeting them.

THE CHANGE PROCESS

In developing a community of learners, a change process was agreed upon by the researchers and the RTO's Flexible Delivery Management Team applying aspects of the work of Boland and Tenaski (1995), which was further developed by Engeström (1999). This is a process whereby systemic tensions and contradictions are reflected back to the team or community, allowing these tensions and contradictions, which the community experiences, to be made visible. The first stage of this process was to interview and observe teachers to gather information about current practices, perspectives, and systemic issues. Findings from this process were then reflected back to the team and used to guide a collaborative design workshop in which changes to teaching strategies were discussed and the parameters mapped for the development of a suitable platform to host ICT resources. Future stages of the project were designed to involve the team members in developing ICT resources and working with these tools, which potentially require different pedagogical practices and understandings.

During this process it was apparent that there was great enthusiasm for the affordances of technologies and greater appreciation of what to some was a shift in pedagogical understandings. This shift in understanding is best explained by illustrating teachers' current pedagogical understandings and skills and confidence with ICT tools.

All team members had been inspired about the possibilities of ICT through participating in a 1-day workshop that focused on learning to use Macromedia Flash and making an instructional video. However, skill and confidence in the use of ICT resources varied significantly, even among the small group of team members. Some team members had used PowerPoint presentations, all used videos and some used a WebCT bank of assessment items with their apprentices. However, the researchers were informed that among the larger team of trades teachers in this department, many were not computer literate, having come from working in industry, generally as contractors, and had not seen a need to use computer technology. In fact, for many, using computers was something to be avoided.

Teachers participating in the project expressed varied degrees of confidence in the use of ICT resources for teaching, particularly with regard to customizing digital resources and providing real work activities. All those involved believed that their objectives for using ICT resources are to teach underpinning knowledge (procedural and some theoretical knowledge), to assist learners to master skills, and to encourage independent learning. However, they were not sure that using ICT resources had anything to do with analysing information, constructing meaning, and organizing ideas and information. This background information helped inform the researchers' development of an intervention strategy. The first step of this strategy was to reflect back to the team what the researchers discovered about current practices and system tensions and contradictions.

Reflecting Back to the Team

What the researchers found and reflected back to the team was that as teachers, they attach paramount importance to the visual, understandably so in trades, where apprentices and skilled workers use visual cues to identify the quality of the work, quality of materials, and possible problems. For this reason, the team emphasized the importance of instructional videos and was intent on making an instructional video for everything, from how to use hand-held tools to putting up roof trusses. Learning as instruction and the teacher as instructor strongly permeated the language of these teachers. Teachers would provide apprentices with information either by working through workbooks with the apprentices, using PowerPoint presentations or demonstrating practical tasks.

While teachers noted that some people are visual learners, some auditory, some tactile, and some are kinesthetic learners, there was puzzlement expressed by a few teachers about why some apprentices pick things up much more quickly than others. Their exposure to the range of different theories of learning styles and types of intelligence was limited. Extending this knowledge would assist these teachers to address puzzles such as this.

A variety of teaching strategies was employed by the team, but most reflected a dominantly instructional, rather than constructivist perspective. Typical teaching strategies included using videos, verbal instruction, demonstration, PowerPoint presentations, and questioning. Teachers reported that typically when using videos they would introduce the title of the video and ask apprentices to watch. The use of videos in this way is consistent with the notion of the teacher as instructor and the apprentices as passive learners. Apprentices were given little reason to focus their attention and there were no explicit expectations of them on completion of the viewing.

Teachers also reported typically asking lots of knowledge and comprehension questions, but mostly closed-ended questions that were only occasionally interspersed with questions requiring higher-order thinking skills. Lower-order knowledge questions such as, "How far down do you place the hinge?" or " What is the spacing between wall studs?", support rote learning, again placing the responsibility for learning with the teacher. The apprentices remain passive learners, not required to fully engage with the content material, to think at a higher level or solve problems.

Typical higher order questions included, "Why? What are the consequences of …? What alternatives are there ….?" and, "How will you…?" Such questions engage the learners, requiring them to take some responsibility. They also acknowledge the ability, experience and knowledge of the apprentices themselves.

One teacher would ask apprentices to draw, for example, a window detail, before fitting a window. This encourages apprentices to think through the detail of what is required and the steps involved. It becomes a check for the tasks they are about to undertake. The responsibility for attending to the detail and ensuring that the required knowledge about how different components go together, becomes that of the individual apprentice, not the teacher.

In a project-based learning environment, higher order questioning, drawing and engagement in practical tasks to develop and demonstrate competency are important and useful strategies. The use of videos, PowerPoint and other ICT resources has the potential to scaffold learning and assist learners in their journey from novice to expert. To move increasingly towards the use of tools and strategies that value and use the developing experience of the apprentices will be a key to the successful implementation of project-based learning through the use of ICT resources. The reflecting back process also involved exploring the tensions between a constructivist project-based approach to learning and flexible delivery, discussed later in the chapter.

The Collective Trajectory in Using ICT Resources

To focus the direction of the efforts being undertaken, it was necessary to agree collectively on the direction of the activity. In reporting and reflecting back to the team, the researchers spoke about flexible delivery. This was quickly re-phrased by the team as flexible learning. Flexible learning was defined by teachers as:

- Being self-paced
- Being outcome rather than time focused
- Developing learning-to-learn skills in apprentices
- Teaching becoming a process of facilitation
- Providing support for learning
- Requiring a variety of resources
- Requiring a variety of learning methods
- Assessing on demand (i.e. when apprentices are ready, rather than at preset times)
- Recognizing that learning occurs at the work-site as well as at the RTO

Given that the decision to develop ICT resources within a project-based learning context was to shape the structures and practices of the team, it is interesting to note the parallels between the above understandings of flexible learning with the pedagogy of project-based learning. For example, the teacher as facilitator, as opposed to instructor, requires teachers to assist students to draw from their own experiences and prior knowledge and integrate new knowledge with existing knowledge (Land and Greene, 2000), as well as to assist learners in analyzing and drawing conclusions, designing, experimenting, making predictions. And above all, to ask questions (Laffey, Tupper, Musser, and Wedman, 1998).

It was also agreed that the desired outcome for apprentices at the completion of their training was an ability to learn. This is another important recognition requiring a shift in pedagogical practice for this team, to one where the teacher facilitates or guides the learner from novice towards becoming an expert in his community (Blanton, Simmons, and Warner, 2001) or industry. This process requires the development of metacognitive (learning-to-learn) skills in learners and it is a radical departure from a predominantly instructional pedagogy. Being clear about the collective direction is important as it keeps the focus on how ICT resources are to be used and for what purpose.

Strategies to Support Project-Based Learning

The Collaborative Design Workshop examined teaching and learning strategies that might facilitate a shift from a predominantly instructional pedagogy towards a more constructivist pedagogy, which is assumed to better match the agreed intentions and trajectory the team has decided upon. One strategy is to use questions, videos, still photographs, and design issues in constructing the learning experiences within the learning platform. Van de Walle (2004) reminds us that learners need multiple ways to think about emerging ideas and knowledge and weave it into a "web of ideas and relational understanding" (p. 30). Therefore multiple approaches are required to provide practice and opportunity to embed newly forming understandings, whether this is accomplished through pictures or real world situations, using oral language, or drawing, for example.

The conflict encountered between an instructional based pedagogy and constructivist pedagogy was evident in a statement made by one participant: "We cannot ask them that [a higher order question] as we have not yet given them the knowledge". The confusion arises from a belief that the only pathway to a satisfactory solution is by way of specific information delivered from a single source. Others in the team felt less dissonance as they began to explore and think differently about learning. This was evident as the team worked with a range of still photographs of doors and windows, some of which were deliberately incorrectly labeled, some were examples of poor practice, and others were typical types of doors or windows. Teachers were asked to develop questions using these photographs as a resource for apprentices. This was an exercise in developing higher order thinking skills and providing practice for teachers to develop skills in asking such questions. One group looking at a photograph where a door was incorrectly labeled as a fire door designed a question asking, 'What is wrong with this picture?' The attempt to ask apprentices to analyse and apply their knowledge of materials required to meet fire safety standards was almost achieved. Although there was laughter about this response, there was a strong sense of support for everyone's attempts to move through the dissonance they were experiencing. A sense of community was evident from within the team.

Using still photographs provides opportunities to compare and contrast and for learners to apply what they already know from experience on the job. For example, instead of asking apprentices a typical question, "How far from the top do you place the hinge to hang a door?", an alternative is to place a scale rule on a series of photographs of different types of doors and ask "What is the same and what is different about how this range of doors is hung?". Such an approach assists in developing apprentices' metacognitive (learning to learn) skills by providing them with the opportunity to develop skills in problem posing and problem solving through a strategy of comparing and contrasting.

While considering the use of still photos and reviewing their own videos members of the team gained insight about the importance of providing the context of the photos and videos for learners viewing these visual resources. Team members themselves experienced confusion when given still photos without the context in which the photos were taken and the purpose for which they might be used. An important aspect of communicative practices for visual communication is to provide the context. For example, a still photo of windows requires a photo of the building in which the windows are situated to assist learners make sense of the visual image. However there are times when teachers may deliberately not provide the context in order to induce thinking about what the typical context might be for the given detail.

The use of videos provides multiple opportunities for using prediction and re-telling. Prediction and re-telling activities draw on apprentices' abilities to clarify their thinking, to connect with what they already know, to organise ideas logically, and to employ higher order cognition, such as inferring and predicting (Cambourne and Turbill, 1987). To successfully use prediction and re-telling, learners need to have been immersed in the language and structure of the content, in this instance, carpentry and joinery skills and competencies. Such activities assume a perception of learning as constructivist, social and collaborative.

Prediction activities explored in the design workshop included stopping the video part way through and asking apprentices to predict what the next step will be or what the outcome of the current step will be. Apprentices are learning to hypothesize the outcomes of a set of actions. Another activity included apprentices working in pairs watching a section of the video with sound track muted while one apprentice (having either seen the video previously or having been introduced to the topic or process being demonstrated in the video) provides his partner the verbal commentary. Roles can then be reversed for the next section. Apprentices can re-wind the video, listen to it, and compare their commentaries with that of the video. Re-telling provides opportunities to use the language of the trade, to develop knowledge of the sequence of tasks, knowledge of quality and how to achieve it, and of course to connect new procedural or conceptual knowledge with existing knowledge, thereby re-ordering or changing cognitive schemas.

Jonassen (2000) reminds us that problem solving, integral to project-based learning, requires an acceptance of uncertainty and the making of judgments. To support learners in this acceptance, it is necessary to attend to the affective domain, creating an environment in which learners feel safe to make attempts, to try a solution and adjust as required (Vella, 2002). Currently, when apprentices are working on the floor at the RTO and undertaking practical tasks such as fitting a bath, swinging a door, building wall frames and so on, there are considerable near attempts and judgments made about what will work and what will not. Teachers support this learning with questions, with demonstration of techniques, and sometimes with redirection. While it is hoped that apprentices will self-evaluate their own work, this does not occur consistently if apprentices have not yet moved out of the role of passive learner in a theory session to active learner in a practical session.

The ICT platform chosen by the group to support the use of videos, text, photographs, questioning, and other activities, is a simple, easy to use and navigate platform, called EXe. During the Collaborative Design Workshop EXe was compared with a quite different platform based on PowerPoint. Teachers explored both and made the following observations about the design principles that need to be considered when developing their own platform:

- The opening page needs to have clear directions and an overview.
- A return to home button is required on every page.
- Help in navigating and accessing the platform needs to be fore- grounded.
- Verbal cues can be added to assist with navigation.
- Where there is audio, control needs to be given to the user to stop, rewind, restart the audio.
- Photos and videos need to take up the whole screen for visual impact and the ability to identify detail.
- Print size needs to be easy to read, larger than 14 point.
- Text should be limited to one message per page.
- Videos, photos, questions, and other activities need to be embedded in a framework.

The general message is to keep the online environment simple, accessible, and easy to use. These teachers and the whole team had previously rejected the complexity of simulated environments, as they are not only expensive and time consuming to develop, but are often difficult to navigate and difficult to keep learners focused. Their intention was to use and design learning in a platform that is accessible and easy to update, thus providing teachers with the ownership of the learning design.

The Collaborative Design Workshop exposed teachers to some different tools to create learning sequences and confronted teachers with difference and dissonance. The supportive community, ownership of the learning platform, and preparedness to try different strategies is important in working through the multiple tensions and contradictions faced by this team.

TENSIONS

Tensions facing this team include:

- Predominantly instruction-based pedagogy versus a need for a constructivist pedagogy .
- A constructivist pedagogy (within a project-based learning environment) requiring collaborative work versus flexible learning where individuals can work individually.

It is clear there is a tension between the predominantly instruction-based pedagogical resources teachers have been using such as workbooks and the more interactive resources required to develop a constructivist learning environment around project-based learning. Project-based learning requires collaborative work, higher order thinking, developing learning-to-learn skills, and generally handing responsibility for learning over to the learners.

Handing over responsibility to students requires a re-thinking of the way tasks and power are distributed between teachers and apprentices. In instruction-based pedagogy, teachers control the pace of learning, including the introduction of new material, and require learners to follow directions and demonstrate expertise. Learners have a passive role. In a constructivist learning pedagogy, learners are active and have some input into what new material is introduced and when. Table 1 lists the roles, that is, the distribution of power and tasks and the rules of engagement, of teachers and apprentices under the different pedagogical approaches.

The use of different resources and tools mediates the roles of teachers and apprentices. A constructivist learning environment requires far more complex and extensive roles of both teachers and learners. Learners take on far more responsibility, while teachers relinquish some of their power and control to encourage learners to take the initiative. The informal, often unspoken rules of engagement in the two different pedagogical practices differ. ICT resources of themselves cannot change practice unless other resources and tools that support the way teachers think about learning and teaching, and the subsequent distribution of power and tasks, and the rules that govern that interaction are also changed.

Table 1. Roles of Teacher and Apprentices

Roles using an instructional pedagogy	
Role of teacher	Role of student
To motivate students	To be told
To provide resources	To follow directions
To be the expert	
To front-end load apprentices with underpinning knowledge	
Roles using a constructivist learning pedagogy	
Identify what learners already know	Have responsibility for self-motivation
Facilitate learning	Develop learning to learn skills
Develop and provide scaffolding to support learning	Predict
Teachers provide and manage resources	Active problem solvers
Coach, provide feedback and encourage	Actively draw on their knowledge and experience
Model skills, behaviors, strategies, techniques, processes	
Challenge the learner	Evaluate their own and others' work

Collaborative versus Individual Learning

The collaborative approach to learning within project-based learning environments is at odds with flexible learning. Flexible learning involves creating approaches to learning and resources where apprentices work individually, at their own pace, rather than collaboratively. This sets up a tension between flexible learning with the learners operating at their own pace and teachers' need to manage learning by keeping some control over the pace of apprentices' formal learning and assessment. It was interesting to note that teachers commented that ICT resources were useful in controlling the pace of apprentices, that is, keeping a group of apprentices at a similar pace as in a traditional classroom approach.

Conclusion

As noted by the Australian Flexible Learning Framework, flexible learning is a change process (ANTA, 2001). Changing teaching practices is more than introducing teachers to ICT resources and developing their skills. Dennen (2005) for example, noted that "tool design may have some effect on pedagogy, but it is the design of specific course activities that affects their ability to generate effective peer and instructor-student interactions." (p. 129).

The change process adopted in this project understands that any system, has inherent tensions and contradictions and that these are more visible when new directions or tools, or rules and task allocation are introduced (Engeström, 1999). To assist the process of making the tensions and contradictions visible, the researchers gathered data about existing practices and reflected these back to the teachers as systemic tensions. The next step was to develop a collective trajectory, and then to develop shared mental models and a common language. The Collaborative Design Workshop was the intervention strategy used to begin this process. Developing shared mental models and a common language takes time, and requires ongoing facilitation. Owen (2001) suggests strategies that assist the development of shared mental models include:

> behaviors such as: asking relevant and thought-provoking questions, sharing observations, seeking alternative perspectives, assertively challenging a particular opinion, seeking clarification and sharing information through processes of consulting and collaborating (p. 598).

Ongoing exchange, discussion and debate are required. As Dennen (2005) stated, ICT resources may have some effect on pedagogy. This is because it creates possibilities. However these possibilities need to be perceived and understood to be used. An ICT learning environment can be constructed just as readily to design an instructional learning experience as it can a constructivist learning experience.

Key to the success of the change program involving the development of new ICT resources and appropriate pedagogies to meet agreed intentions is that teachers have direct control of the design and content of the tools they are producing. The decision to reject complex ICT resources developed by others ensures ownership and a continuing ability to readily update materials, such as photos and videos where the content may quickly become out of date as building technologies change.

One of the many challenges facing this team is the extent to which the team will use the ICT resources they develop as stand-alone resources, or as part of an integrated process of teaching and learning practices for flexible learning. Researchers will work with the team in the continuing stages of the project to facilitate ongoing exchange, discussion and debate. We will provide material and content for such exchange by undertaking an analysis of the communicative practices of the ICT resources developed by the team and observing teachers and apprentices using them. This will assist the team to continuously evaluate their work and address questions such as:

- What is needed to support apprentices in inducting them into the use of these resources?
- How to support students to develop their metacognitive skills, especially if there is greater expectations for students to work more independently.
- How to modify and update the resource to ensure optimal communication?
- What understandings and skills do teachers need in order to further develop their instructional design skills?
- What understandings and skills do teachers need in order to further develop their ICT pedagogy?

REFERENCES

ANTA. (1998). *Eyes wide open - vocational education and training in the information age.* Brisbane: Author.

ANTA. (2001). *Shaping our Future. Australia's national strategy for vocational education and training 2004-2010.* Brisbane: Author.

Blanton, W., Simmons, E., and Warner, M. (2001). The Fifth Dimension: Application of cultural-historical activity theory, inquiry-based learning, computers, and telecommunications to change prospective teachers' preconceptions. *Journal Educational Computing Research, 24*, 435-463.

Boland, R., and Tenaski, R. (1995). Perspective making and perspective taking in communities of knowing. *Organization Science, 6*, 350-372.

Cambourne, B., and Turbill, J. (1987). *Coping with Chaos.* Rozelle, NSW, Australia: Primary English Teaching Association.

Dennen, V. (2005). From Message Posting to Learning Dialogues: Factors affecting learner participation in asynchronous discussion. *Distance Education, 26*, 127-148.

Engestrom, Y. (1999). Expansive visibilization of work: An activity -theoretical perceptive. *Computer Supported Cooperative Work, 8*, 63-93.

Jonassen, D. (2000). Toward a Design Theory of Problem Solving. *ETRandD, 48*, 63-85.

Kilpatrick, S., and Bound, H. (2003). *Learning Online: Benefits and barriers in regional Australia - Volume 1.* Adelaide: NCVER.

Laffey, J., Tupper, T., Musser, D., and Wedman, J. (1998). A Computer-Mediated Support System for Project-Based Learning. *Educational Technology, Research and Development, 46*, 73-86.

Land, S., and Greene, B. (2000). Project-Based Learning with the World Wide Web: A qualitative study of resource integration. *Educational Technology, Research and Development, 48*, 45-67.

Owen, C. (2001). The role of organisational context in mediating workplace learning and performance. *Computers in Human Behavior, 17*, 597-614.

Van de Walle, J. (2004). *Elementary and middle school mathematics teaching developmentally*. Boston: Pearson Education.

Vella, J. (2002). *Learning to Listen: Learning to Teach: The power of dialogue in educating adults*. New York: John Wiley and Sons.

In: New Research in Education Adult, Medical and Vocational ISBN 978-1-60741-873-3
Editors: Edmondo Balistrieri and Giustino DeNino © 2009 Nova Science Publishers, Inc.

Chapter 6

TURNING UP THE VOLUME: YOUNG ADULTS REFLECT ON THEIR SECONDARY SCHOOL EXPERIENCE*

Deborah Espiner[1],† and Diane Guild[2]
[1]Faculty of Education, University of Auckland, New Zealand
[2]Professional Development and Outreach Services, Mt. Richmond Special School, Auckland, New Zealand

ABSTRACT

The "voice" of students with disabilities typically goes unheard. Valuable insights to strengthen academic and social learning are missed when students are not consulted with or listened to. This chapter describes the use of graphic facilitation to capture the voice of a group of four young adults with special educational needs. Participation in a conference presentation enabled them to share personal ideas about their secondary school experiences with a group of special educators. The special educators who observed the process found that it was an effective way to hear and capture the student voice. It provided them with valuable insights and information for the ongoing development of the meaningful and supportive educational programmes in secondary schools. Listening to the voice of young people and involving them in the design of the educational experience will turn up the volume to ensure that the voice fashions the educational journey.

INTRODUCTION

This chapter focuses on a group of four young adults with special educational needs who volunteered to participate in a conference presentation in which they were asked to reflect on

---

* A version of this chapter was also published in *Challenging Thinking about Teaching and Learning*, edited by C.M. Rubie-Davies and C. R published by Nova Science Publishers, Inc. It was submitted for appropriate modifications in an effort to encourage wider dissemination of research.

† Correspondence regarding this chapter should be addressed by email to: debbie.espiner@auckland.ac.nz.

and share their thoughts about their secondary school experiences. The presentation was observed by a group of special educators.

There were three purposes to this presentation. The first was to provide a forum in which the young adults could share their ideas and feelings about their time at secondary school. This would include ways in which the secondary school experience could have been improved for them. The second purpose was to enable the observers to better understand the perspectives of the young adults, through the use of graphic facilitation to increase the observers' engagement with the ideas expressed by the young adults. The third purpose was to demonstrate a process that helped to elicit these ideas and feelings and enabled the observers to really hear what the young adults were saying.

LITERATURE REVIEW

New Zealand is striving to be a more inclusive society. This is the central purpose of the New Zealand Disability Strategy (Minister for Disability Issues, 2001), which provides a framework for increasing the awareness of and responding to the needs of disabled people. To develop a more inclusive society, the New Zealand Disability Strategy advocates recognition of disabled people as "experts on their own experience" (p. 14), which means ensuring that "disabled people are asked what they think" (Ministry of Health, 2001, p. 4). Inclusion will be achieved by eliminating barriers that disabled people may experience when participating in and contributing to society.

Since the 1989 New Zealand Education Act, there has been a focus on increasing the presence and participation of students with disabilities in their local schools. Education provision in New Zealand ranges from regular schools to settings that are highly specialized. The degree of inclusion depends on the climate, attitudes, knowledge, skills, and resources of the school community. The ability of the school to "tune into" and hear the student voice will influence students' presence and participation.

An inclusive school meets the needs of all students through equitable funding, policies, processes, and practices (Booth and Ainscow, 2002; Slee, 2001). Students also must take a full and active part in, and be valued members of, the school community (Fraser, 2005; Nakken and Pijl, 2002). A study in the United Kingdom (Department for Education and Skills, 2001) set out to determine how services delivered by government departments affected children and young people and how children and young people could be involved in developing more inclusive practices. The report reinforces the concept that when students take a role in the decision making at school, practices improve and school citizenship is promoted (Department for Education and Skills, 2001). This report advocates making the shift from assuming "we know best, towards putting those whose lives we affect in the driving seat" (p. 3). Objective 5 in the New Zealand Disability Strategy recognizes the "driving seat" by advocating leadership through a specific action to "encourage disabled people to take part in decision-making as service users . . . within all services that disabled people access" (Minister for Disability Issues, 2001, 5.1, p. 19).

Objective 3 in the New Zealand Disability Strategy lists actions that contribute to providing quality education for disabled people. This includes ensuring that all those involved in education and social services understand the learning needs of disabled people by acknowledging and acting on their ideas, thoughts, and feelings. This is also reflected in the National Administration Guidelines (Ministry of Education, 2007), which require schools to be responsive to and accountable for these needs.

Processes and strategies for involving students in decision making must be explored and developed. The voice of young people is often overlooked, not listened to, or not acted upon. The New Zealand Education Review Office (ERO) reported that the promotion of student participation in decision making is an area for further development:

The participation of students with special needs in school decision-making was predominantly limited to input at a classroom level, mainly into individual learning programmes. Schools need to ensure that students with special needs are provided with real opportunities, matched to student abilities, to participate in school decision-making. (ERO, 2003, pp. 13–14)

Creating opportunities for students to have input into decision making will influence what happens to and around them. The "absent voices of students with disabilities is of particular concern, since their right to be consulted and have a say in decisions affecting their lives is enshrined in current rights-based policy" (Bray and Gates, 2000 p. 58). Ways of sharing experiences and engaging with what is being said will lead to more responsive person-focused approaches to service provision. It is well documented that people have different processing and learning styles (Gardner, 1985; Armstrong, 1987). In order to engage students to the fullest extent, it is important to capitalize on the full range of learning styles rather than focusing primarily on the traditional verbal–linguistic ones.

To increase both engagement with content and interaction with participants, visual techniques are being promoted (Caldwell, Dake, Safly, and Ulch, 2000). Horn (1998) states that visual–verbal language enhances the quality of communication and that combining visual and verbal modes is more effective than words alone. Mayer (2001) supports adding visuals to words and the use of visual–verbal "stand-alone" diagrams. Tierney (2003) supports this, claiming that people retain 10% of information they read, 20% of information they hear, and 50% of information they see and hear.

According to Woolsey (1996), visual communication enables people to concentrate on ideas under discussion and build a framework of shared understanding and learning. People can more quickly integrate and act on information that has been recorded visually (Clegg, 2003; Horn, 1998). The use of visual techniques is also an effective way of disseminating large amounts of information and enabling more collaborative and effective dialogue (Horn, 1998).

Visual language is a growing area that illustrates the effectiveness of using graphics, text, and pictures (Horn, 1998). One process that assists the development of dialogue and understanding through visual–verbal channels is graphic facilitation (Sibbett, 1981). As the name suggests, graphic facilitation has two main components—facilitation and graphic recording. Ideally, two facilitators work with a group—a process facilitator who draws out ideas, issues and themes, and a graphic recorder who captures the ideas expressed by the individual or developed by the group. Ideas are recorded on a large chart in full view of everyone participating. The chart provides a canvas on which the visual dialogue develops. This enables specific details to be recorded while at the same time presenting the "big picture".

Kim and Mauborgne (2002) believe that building the process around a picture creates much better results than using the traditional written format. Furthermore, the chart provides a vehicle for thinking together and capturing and linking multiple perspectives. The resulting graphic contains large amounts of information that can be understood at a glance. Horn (1998) discusses the visual mapping of ideas through the creation of information landscapes (p. 95). He states this type of communication format lends itself well "to broad, systems-level overviews of complex situations or ideas" (p. 63). Furthermore, the use of a large chart enables specifics and details to be recorded and linkages between ideas made apparent as they "positively affect" how we communicate "big ideas." (p. 63).

In addition to stimulating new meaning and insight, the graphic also serves as a group memory for reflection and further development. Sibbett refers to graphic facilitation as "public listening". He claims that participants in a meeting immediately see ideas captured and reframed—making it possible for them to clarify their thoughts. Ownership of the dialogue is enhanced through the participants' identification with the graphics as they are recorded.

THE STUDY

The purpose of the conference presentation was threefold: to provide a context in which young adults (the participants) would feel comfortable expressing their ideas; to provide a context where professionals (the observers) could hear and reflect on the young adults' voices; and to demonstrate a process known to engage both speakers and listeners.

Methodology

The method therefore needed to do more than merely engage the participants in a conversation. The investigation was not designed purely to "survey the terrain" (McCracken, 1988, p. 17) or to conduct an overview, but to "mine it" (McCracken, 1988, p. 17)—to obtain a deeper understanding of individual perspectives and the relationships between them. It was hoped that the combined techniques of focused conversation (Clough and Nutbrown, 2003) and graphic facilitation (Sibbett,1981) would be useful tools for capturing the voices, experiences, stories, new expressions, and new learning in a shared dynamic of communication (Clough and Nutbrown, 2002) that provided both big picture and detail.

Elements of the focus group approach (Merton and Kendall, 1946) also supported the investigation in the way that it enabled a structured dialogue to develop around a chosen topic. It allowed participants "to prompt as well as to 'bounce' ideas off one another" (Waldegrave, 2003, p. 251) and produced "considerable and often complex information in a comparatively short space of time" (Alice, 2003, p. 64). The process encouraged participants to express ideas, values, and beliefs in their own language, highlighting their view of the world (Kitzinger, 1994). Morgan and Krueger (1993) write of the importance of this technique especially when there are power differences between participants and professionals.

The method reflected elements of a focused conversation in the way it elicited the voices of a smaller group of people, exploring how their collective experiences fitted together. The technique of the focused conversation has similar advantages to those of the focus group. Both techniques capitalize on synergism, snowballing, stimulation, security, and spontaneity

(Hess, 1968). The key difference between the two techniques is that a focus group typically involves answering a set of questions whereas the focused conversation often raises, rather than answers, questions (Clough and Nutbrown, 2002). As the purpose of the presentation was to capture the voice of the young adults (who had recently left school), it was important that space and freedom be provided to enable the conversation to be directed by them.

Participants

To achieve the intended purpose of the presentation, it was important that the participants were young adults with disabilities who had left school in the last two to three years and who were previously unknown to the researchers. The time frame was relevant to the investigation in that it provided the balance of a distance from the schooling experience while maintaining a recent perspective. A group of four young adults with special educational needs participated to share personal ideas about their secondary school experiences with a group of special educators.

Procedure

In selecting participants, the researchers enlisted the assistance of a person who facilitates regular support meetings of young people with disabilities and their caregivers. The opportunity to participate in this conference presentation and research was discussed at one of the regular fortnightly meetings. Four young adults, two women and two men between the ages of 18 and 23 years, volunteered to participate. All had left school within the past two to three years.

On receiving names and contact details of the participants, the researchers contacted them and their parents. The presentation, the research project, and the practical details were discussed. Information sheets and consent forms were then mailed out to participants and their parents.

Before the presentation, there was an opportunity for the participants to reacquaint with one another and to meet the facilitators. There was also an opportunity to review the process and clarify uncertainties. It was considered vital that every effort be made to put the participants at ease. In a similar way, immediately after the presentation the young adults met with the facilitators for a debriefing on the experience.

For the presentation, participants sat in a semicircle side-on to the observers. This limited eye contact between participants and observers, provided maximum eye contact between participants and facilitators, and enabled everyone to view the evolving graphic.

At the outset of the session, the facilitators explained to the observers the structure of the presentation and the procedure that would be followed. An evaluation form was distributed to observers, who were invited to complete it at the conclusion of the presentation. The evaluation form required observers to reflect, rank, and comment on the process used to elicit participants' voices. The form consisted of four questions that required respondents to provide a ranking on a five-point scale and invited them to make additional comments if they wished.

The facilitators introduced themselves and then invited each participant to introduce him or herself. Three key questions and a number of prompts were used to guide the discussion. Each participant in turn contributed responses relating to what they considered was good about secondary school, what was helpful, and what would have made secondary school better.

A template had been pre-drawn providing the three key words (good, helpful, and better) to provide structure for the participants and to reinforce the direction of the discussion. This template was referred to as a "schoolscape" to convey the idea of developing a "landscape" of participants' ideas (see Figure 1).

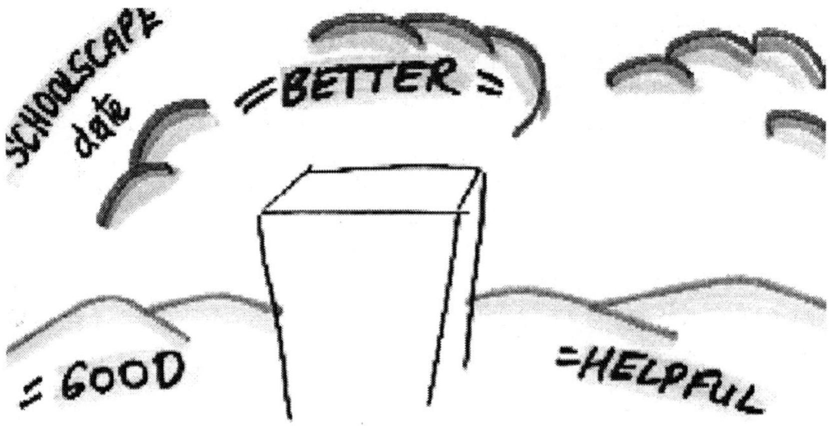

Figure 1. Template of the Schoolscape.

The feelings and ideas of each participant were recorded in a different colour to enable observers to identify and track individual participants' contributions and to assist with analysis of content after the presentation.

Introductions were recorded in the school building in the centre of the graphic. This provided the focal point for all further dialogue. The graphic developed as each segment was introduced and each participant responded. Responses to the questions relating to what participants felt was "good" about secondary school and what they found "helpful" were recorded on the land of the schoolscape. This grounded the discussion and provided a foundation for the next segment, which focused on what would have made school better. These responses were recorded in the sky to represent new ways of doing things, dreams and the winds of change.

Results

The following discussion is divided into three parts. The first part unpacks the schoolscape (illustrated in full in Figure 2) which highlights the voices of the young people—the participants. This covers the introduction to the participants (Figure 3), the discussion on what was good about school (Figure 4), the discussion of what was most helpful for the young people while they were at school (Figure 5), and discussion of what could have been better (Figure 6). The second part presents the findings collated from the evaluation forms that observers completed at the conclusion of the presentation. The third part presents comments made by the young people in the debriefing session that followed the presentation.

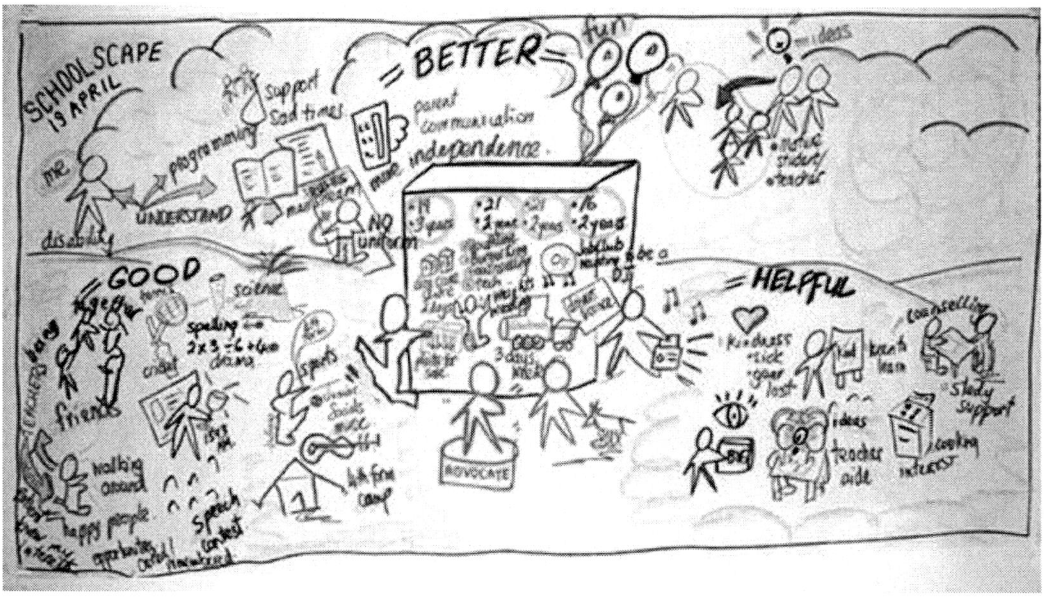

Figure 2. The Completed Schoolscape.

The Voices of the Participants

Introductions

The participants were invited to introduce themselves. They were asked to indicate the time lapse since they left secondary school and to talk about their interests, as recorded below (see also Figure 3):

Phillip was 21 when he left school two years ago. His ambition is to become a DJ in a night club. This ambition he attributes to his passion for music and self-confidence he feels he gained through participating in speech competitions at school. Phillip is currently training in wrestling and weight lifting.

Taylor is 18—he left school two years ago. Taylor is very interested and informed about trains. He knows the distinguishing features and functions of a variety of trains. He works at Glenbrook Vintage Railway three days a week. Taylor has his Learner's (driving) Licence and is currently working towards his Restricted Licence. He also has an interest in music having auditioned for and competed in New Zealand Idol.

Bronwyn left school three years ago—she is now 22. She is attending a technical institute, has a part-time job at Burger King and is training to be a Youthline phone counsellor. In addition to her interest in counselling, Bronwyn has an ambition to be a spokesperson and advocate for people with disabilities. She is aware of a range of disabilities and is very informed about her own specific disability. Bronwyn is concerned about the implications of having a disability in today's society.

Laura is now 23, having left school two years ago. Laura's interests are in the field of nurturing. She is currently working in a day care centre two days a week. With family support, Laura is developing a boutique business raising plants from seedlings. She is currently restoring glasshouses to plant in readiness for the Christmas market. Laura also enjoys working and being with animals.

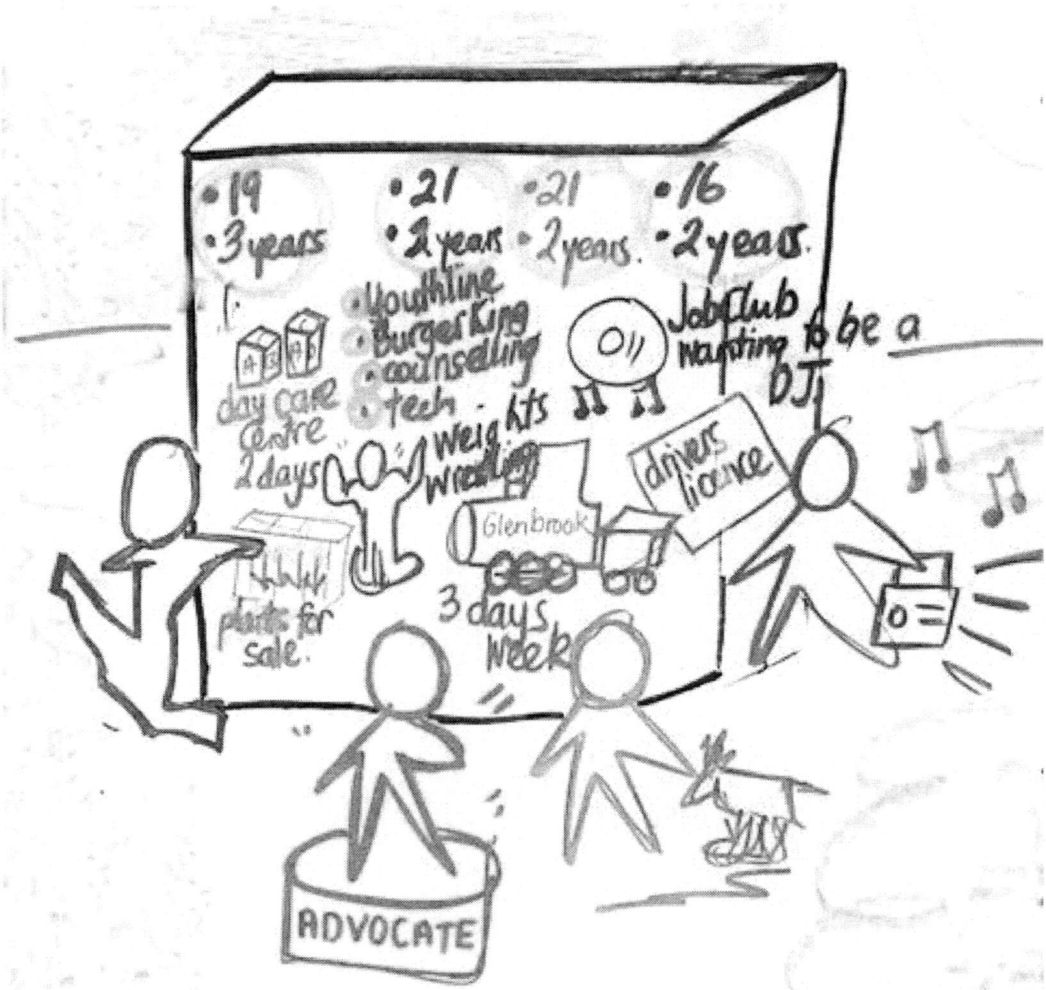

Figure 3. Introductions.

Each of the four participants was well connected to the community through work and interest pursuits. They had a number of interests and were very clear about their ambitions for ongoing personal development. This provided a basis and an impetus to discuss and reflect on their secondary schooling. It is interesting that although some of these participants had been supported by a special unit, they had all attended a regular secondary school. This may be a contributing factor for their post-school success, as regular school involvement enhances transition into adulthood and promotes wider community involvement and develops career skills (Sax, Noyes, and Fisher, 2001; Carubba, 1998; DiGiacomo, 2002, as cited in MacArthur, Kelly, and Higgins, 2005). Making the transition to adult life and connecting with the wider community is often seen as the "litmus test" of the quality of the school experience (MacArthur, Kelly, and Higgins, 2005, p. 57).

What Was Good About School?

There were five or six common factors identified by each of the participants as being the key to their enjoyment of secondary school (see Figure 4). They were all related to the importance of belonging—the sense of community that the participants experienced through social contacts and being linked to the wider school. All the participants had enjoyed opportunities to participate in a range of school-wide activities. These included social events, school camps, speech competitions, and sports events. Having opportunities to discover and develop new skills also featured as important.

The development of relationships appeared to be the most highly valued factor that contributed to participants' enjoyment. They all expressed an appreciation of teachers remembering them and taking an interest in their well-being and academic progress. The importance of relationships in an educational context is well documented in the literature and recognized as being a key factor in the development of social competence and self esteem (Meyer and Bevan-Brown, 2005). Over the past decade, a number of New Zealand research programmes (Alton-Lee, 2003; Hill and Hawke, 2001; Bishop, Berryman, Richardson, and Tiakiwai, 2003; Ministry of Education, 2004) have further demonstrated the importance of relationships in a variety of educational settings.

The following summaries, to be read in conjunction with Figure 4, capture the participants' views on what was good about school:

Phillip's secondary schooling was supported through his placement in a unit for students with learning disabilities. This gave him the support he needed in order to participate in school speech competitions. Phillip particularly enjoyed the opportunities to develop friendships in this setting. He appreciated when people noticed, "cared and remembered" him.

Laura enjoyed academic subjects. She mentioned spelling and maths as being particularly enjoyable. Secondary schooling provided her with opportunities to participate in a range of sporting activities. Laura especially enjoyed playing tennis and cricket.

Bronwyn enjoyed being part of the school community. She enjoyed "walking around the school [and being among] happy people". Bronwyn commented that even when she was not directly involved with a group she still felt she belonged. Bronwyn enjoyed interacting with teachers and the interest they showed in her. Science was Bronwyn's favourite subject, particularly the work she did on volcanoes.

Taylor enjoyed his fourth form year the best. He felt that by this time he had learned to find his way around the school and how to interact in the secondary setting. His fourth form recollections included going to school camp and participating in sports. Taylor enjoyed the socials and felt they had provided great opportunities for his musical expression. He appreciated the time teachers took to get to know him and his interests. He felt that they were patient and created opportunities for him to experience a range of activities and develop his strengths.

What was Most Helpful While at School?

The second question, "What was most helpful while at school?", explored what had been helpful in assisting the participants at secondary school (see Figure 5). It was explained to participants that, at the time, they may not have enjoyed or appreciated these aspects but on reflection they realized these had been helpful in their ongoing development. The following summarizes the participants' views.

Bronwyn found the counselling services at school helpful. She also found the kindness of teachers and classmates helpful especially when she felt unwell or had lost some of her gear.

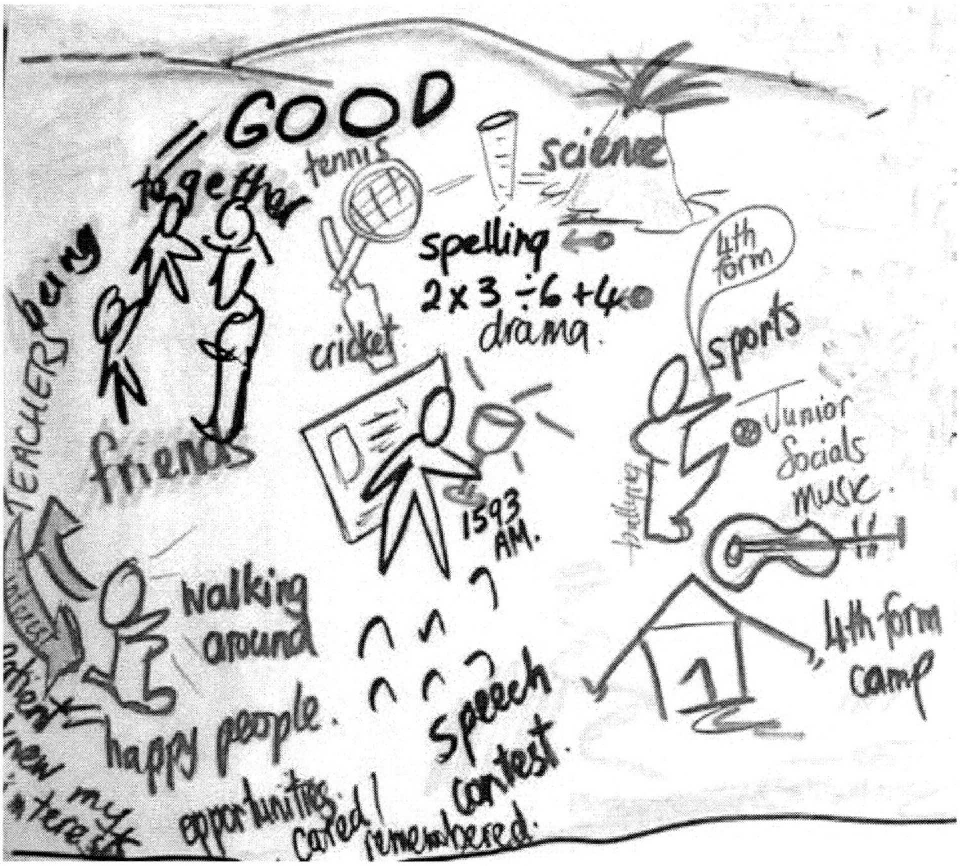

Figure 4. What Was Good about School?

Taylor remembered it had been helpful to have support with developing study skills. Being in the unit provided him with support to complete work he was studying in mainstream classes. He found the opportunities to develop practical skills like cooking particularly helpful.

Phillip talked about the importance and value of teachers keeping a "big picture—seeing me as a whole person" when designing learning activities and opportunities.

Laura recalled how helpful it had been when teachers were kind and keen to help her to learn. She remembered in particular her work with teacher aides. Laura found it helpful having the support of teacher aides who asked her questions and worked through problems with her rather than just telling her what to do.

The common theme in the responses was the support the participants had experienced. This support was evident in a variety of forms; for example, counselling, learning how to study, completing work, and developing practical skills.

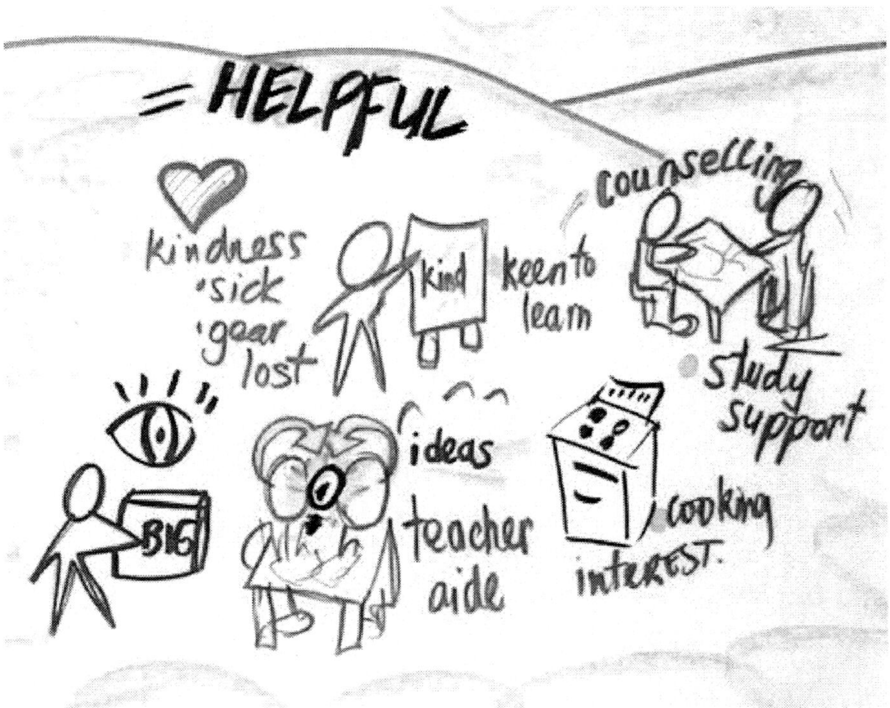

Figure 5. What Was Most Helpful While at School?

Phillip's appreciation of teachers' recognition of the importance of the "whole" person and their taking into account students' interests and strengths demonstrates the value of having education programmes tailored to specific needs and aspirations. The group agreed with this. They also agreed with Laura when she talked about how helpful it had been when teacher aides worked with her to brainstorm and problem solve rather than just giving her the answers. This they found to be a more exciting and meaningful way of learning. The role of the teacher aide is pivotal in the education of students with special educational needs. It is an important and challenging role and New Zealand research recognizes the complex and skilled role teacher aides are expected to undertake in regular classrooms, often without adequate support or training (MacArthur, Kelly, and Higgins, 2005).

What Could Have Been Better?

The common themes identified through the third question, "What could have been better?", present a challenge for teachers and professionals who support students with special needs in secondary schools. The participants' views are given below:

Bronwyn wished people had shown a greater understanding of her disability and the implications this had on her learning. She said it would have helped to have "teachers understanding my learning needs and developing programmes that would help me learn in the mainstream". Bronwyn also commented that "regular communication [by the school] with my parents" would have made secondary school better.

Phillip commented that the only thing that might have enhanced his secondary school experience was "more support at school in times when I was feeling sad".

Taylor wanted "more independence" at secondary school. His suggestions included students "having more say in the rules" and not having to wear a uniform. Considerable discussion and whole group agreement followed Taylor's suggestion that, when they started in the third form, it would have been helpful to "have an older student for a buddy. Someone to give me ideas and show me how to be part of the group—how to behave. Someone to be a friend and help me make friends". He suggested this person needed to be "mature" and have a recognized status "like a head prefect or captain of a sports team".

Laura agreed with all these ideas and indicated she had nothing further to add.

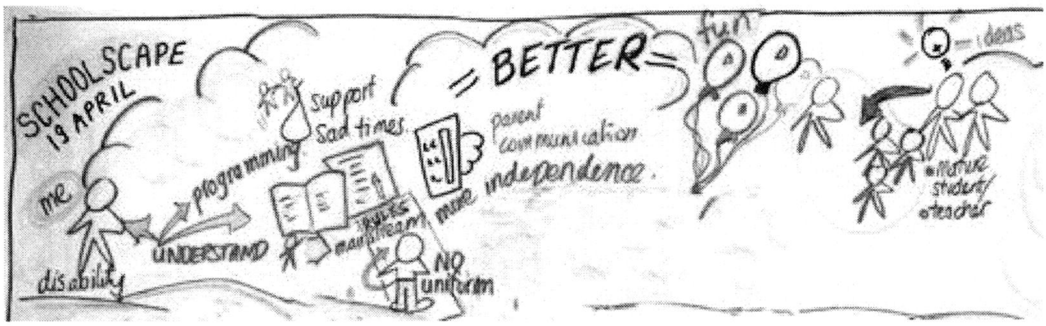

Figure 6. What Could Have Been Better?

The findings (see Figure 6) clearly indicate the importance of teachers getting to know their students, understanding their disabilities, recognizing the implications of these in the learning and social contexts and being able to take them into account when planning programmes. Teachers need to know students well enough to be able to recognize when they are feeling sad and to provide appropriate support. Regular communication with parents would, as Bronwyn recognized, also assist teachers to be more knowledgeable about and understanding of their students (Fraser, 2005).

There is also potential for fostering and further developing peer support systems in secondary schools. In answering previous questions, all the participants identified the importance of the various forms of support they had received. Taylor's concept of having an older "friend" who would be a positive role model and social skills coach from the beginning of secondary school appealed to the group. Developing positive peer cultures in which young people encourage and support each other is a more effective and encompassing approach (Brendtro and Shahbazian, 2004). When Taylor spoke of wanting more independence by having a say in school rules and not wearing a school uniform, he was identifying the fundamental need students have for power, independence, and decision making in the school context. Positive peer cultures provide numerous opportunities to satisfy this need. Features of a positive peer culture include collaborative problem solving, the creation of safe environments, and the development of interpersonal skills through interacting with older peers who are positive role models. The advantage of such an approach would see secondary schools become more like learning organisations embedded in a culture of positive support rather than pockets of support that is dependent on individuals.

Findings from the Observers' Evaluation Forms

Twenty-one of the 33 observers completed an evaluation form. Almost all qualified their rankings with comments in most sections.

The first question asked observers to indicate how helpful observing this process had been in assisting them to identify possible areas for further development in their professional practice. Responses ranged from helpful to extremely helpful (see Table 1, Question 1).

Observers' comments indicated that the process had enabled them to identify possible areas for further development in supporting secondary schools to be more responsive to the needs of students. A range of areas was identified where further support and more effective strategies could be developed. Some of these included social relationships, self-determination, levels of support, inclusive programming, and the lived experience of disability. The importance of listening for the "voice" of the young person was also highlighted in comments that indicated recognition of "the need to ask young people what helps, what is needed and what they think about their school programme".

Other comments reflected how the process had increased observers' understanding and ability to empathize with young people. These comments included that "it gave a real insight into how young people feel about school" and that the conversation "was not as focused on curriculum but more on social (aspects) and being involved in decision making". The process demonstrated to observers that "young people can be involved in decision making about their lives and their future".

The second question asked observers how thought provoking they had found the process. All responses provided a ranking between "thought provoking" and "extremely thought provoking" with a marked number at the higher end of the continuum—82% of observers ranked the process as either very or extremely thought provoking (see Table 1, Question 2).

Observers' comments in this section highlighted the way the process had engaged them and enabled them to identify with what the participants said and how they felt. They reported that the process "gave some insight into how varying disabilities are dealt with in the secondary environment" and that to "see a different side to the story is good". Other comments stated that observers had "loved it as it made it real" and "that it was good to hear first hand". One observer commented that the process "made me really think" and another that the technique was "very welcome at a conference such as this". Responses to both these questions demonstrate Sibbett's (1981) theory that graphic facilitation increases understanding through visual–verbal channels.

When asked to rate the facilitation of the process, most respondents indicated they found it to be either very good (20%) or excellent (65%) (see Table 1, Question 3). Positive feedback was given about the teamwork demonstrated by the two facilitators and about "the balanced approach". Responses included statements such as the process was "very appropriate . . . well thought through . . . extremely special to be here" and "it will be very memorable". This highlighted an important requirement of effective graphic facilitation—the dynamic between the two facilitators as they share the task of developing the process. One, the process facilitator, has the responsibility of building the connection and relationship with and between the participants and encouraging them to share their ideas. The other, the graphic facilitator, concentrates on capturing, organising, and recording the ideas in a meaningful visual language. At the end of each segment, the graphic facilitator checked the accuracy of the graphic by reporting back to the group.

The effectiveness of the process was further affirmed by responses to the fourth question that invited feedback on how helpful it had been for observers to see a discussion recorded in this way. The majority of respondents found it to be a most or very helpful technique (see Table 1, Question 4).

Table 1. Summary of Results

Questions	Ranking and number (%)				
How helpful was this process for identifying possible areas for further development in professional practice	Not helpful	Somewhat helpful	Helpful	Very helpful	Extremely helpful
	0	0	33	19	48
How thought provoking was this experience?	Not very	A little	Thought provoking	Very	Extremely
	0	0	19	19	62
How did you find the facilitation of the process?	Poor	Fair	Good	Very good	Excellent
	0	0	15	20	65
How helpful was it to see the discussion recorded in this way?	Not helpful	Somewhat helpful	Quite helpful	Most helpful	Very helpful
	0	0	14	28.5	57.5

A number of comments drew attention to the power of the visuals alongside the facilitation process. Observers stated that such a technique "allowed for a great deal of honesty on the part of the participants" and that it was "great to hear the students' views first hand". They specifically mentioned how much they "loved the visual graphic process" and that "it helped [us] to have a visual idea of what was said". One observer said that "as I have a hearing impairment, it reinforced what I was hearing" and another commented on the usefulness of the feedback at the end of each section as this provided both a clarification and a summary. Several respondents focused on the power of the graphic message and the building up of the template.

Overall, observers indicated the process had highlighted "the frailties and difficulties students faced whilst at secondary school" and that it had demonstrated "the keenness, characters, and courage of the young people" who had participated. The participants' "awareness of their disabilities and how articulate they were in conveying their thoughts" also impressed observers. Remarks included reference to the participants "openness and willingness to share ideas", their "insights", and how "confident and communicative they [the participants] were". "The wonderful attitude and passion [the participants have] for their interests and for life in general" also impressed the observers.

It was obvious by these and other comments that observers had learned "about the frustrations and experiences of students with special needs in school settings", about "the sort of support and intervention that can truly benefit students with disabilities" and about "the different levels of support [needed]—as perceived by participants".

Observers' comments portrayed how impressed they were with the way, "despite blocks and difficulties being put in their way", participants had "positive attitudes towards past endeavours and personal growth" and how the young people could reframe "negative experiences and integrate them into positive learning".

The Debriefing

The participants' positive attitudes commented on by the observers was evident at the conclusion of the presentation. The young adults who participated in this experience were elated. While they felt relieved that the presentation was over, they were also excited about how "great it had been". Naturally, they had been a little apprehensive about talking in front of teachers and sharing their feelings about "how school could be made better". At the same time they recognized the importance of what they had shared. They said they felt proud that they had been able "to teach the teachers". The participants commented that they enjoyed doing this together. They felt supported in the group context and the quieter participants found it easier to speak up once others had spoken.

Seeing their ideas expressed in the colourful graphics was affirming as they realized their ideas were being heard. They all asked if they could do this again. Their celebration of the event continued in more informal chatter in the car on the way home.

Conclusion

Kim and Mauborgne (2002) challenge facilitators, when they encounter a complex communication problem, to use graphic facilitation. "Listening to subjects with special educational needs throws into a particular relief all the generically difficult issues of researching voice" (Clough and Nutbrown, 2003, p. 71). The process of graphic facilitation is one way of levelling the inevitable imbalance of power between the researcher and the researched—particularly in a special educational context. In the situation described here, the combination of graphic facilitation and focused conversation techniques proved to be very effective in "turning up the volume on the depressed or inaudible voice" (Clough and Nutbrown, 2003, p. 71). This approach supported the young adults to express their ideas and opinions in front of a group of professionals who were vested with the responsibility of designing and implementing educational programmes, supports, and processes for young people with special educational needs. The "engaged" professionals discovered areas for future development in their own professional practice.

The process worked synergistically. It did more than merely engage the young adults in a conversation. It mined the depths of the young adults' perspectives (McCracken, 1988) by creating a context in which the voices of the young adults were heard. The process gave the professionals insights, made it real, made the professionals think, and presented a different perspective. The essence of the participants' voices was captured in a deeper and more meaningful way providing a "whole" as well as the parts—the specifics as well as the big picture.

Giving the lead to the lived experience of disability by listening to the voice of young people and involving them in the design of the educational experience will turn up the volume to ensure that the voice fashions the educational journey.

REFERENCES

Alice, L. (2003). Power, experience and process in feminist research. In C. Davidson, and M. Tolich (Eds.). *Social science research in New Zealand* (2nd ed.).(pp. 61–68). Auckland, New Zealand: Pearson.

Alton-Lee, A. (2003). *Quality teaching for diverse students: Best evidence synthesis.* Wellington, New Zealand: Ministry of Education, Medium Term Strategy Division.

Armstrong, T. (1987). *In their own way.* New York: Tarcher Press.

Bishop, R., Berryman, M., Richardson, C., and Tiakiwai, S. (2003). *Te kotahitanga: The experiences of Year 9 and 10 Maori students in mainstream classrooms.* Hamilton, New Zealand: Maori Education Research Unit (MERU), University of Waikato.

Booth, T., and Ainscow, M. (2002). *The index for inclusion: Developing learning and participation in schools.* Bristol, UK: Centre for Studies on Inclusive Education.

Bray, A., and Gates, S. (2000). Children with disabilities: Equal rights or different rights? In A. Smith, M. Gollop, K. Marshall and K. Nairn (Eds.), *Advocating for children: International Perspectives on Children's Rights,* pp. 32-41. Dunedin, New Zealand: University of Otago Press.

Brendtro, L., and Shahbazian, M. (2004). Troubled Children and Youth: *Turning problems into opportunities.* IL: Research Press.

Caldwell, B., Dake, D., Safly, M., and Ulch, L. (1999–2000). *Brain based visual education.* Iowa State University, IA. Retrieved 11 April, http://www.public.iastate.edu /~design/ ART/NAB/brain4.html.

Clegg, E. (2003). Visual learning: Building knowledge, innovation and collaboration. *Global Learning Resources, 3*(2). Retrieved August 14, 2006 from http://www.glresources.com.

Clough, P. and Nutbrown, C. (2002). *A student's guide to methodology.* London: Sage.

Department of Education and Skills. (2001). *Learning to listen: Core principles for the involvement of children and young people.* Available from www.dfes.gov.uk/ listeningtolearn.

Educational Review Office (ERO). (2003). *Student participation in school decision-making.* Available from http://www.ero.govt.nz/ ero/publishing.nsf/Content/Student%20 Participation% 20in%20School%20Decision-Making.

Fraser, D. (2005). Collaborating with parents/caregivers and whanau. In D. Fraser, R Moltzen, and K. Ryba (Eds.), *Learners with Special Needs in Aotearoa New Zealand* (pp. 128–154). Palmerston North, New Zealand: Thomson Press.

Gardner, H. (1985). *Frames of mind: Theory of multiple intelligences.* New York: Basic Books.

Hess, J. M. (1968). Group interviewing. In R. L. King (Ed.), *New science of planning* (pp. 51–84). Chicago: American Marketing Association.

Hill, J., and Hawke, K. (2001). *Towards making achievement cool: Achievement in multi cultural high schools* (AIMHI). Wellington, New Zealand: Ministry of Education.

Horn, R. E. (1998). *Visual language: Global communication for the 21st century.* Bainbridge Island, New Zealand: MacroVU Press.

Kim, W. C., and Mauborgne, R. (2002, June). Charting your company's future. *Harvard Business Review,* pp. 77–83.

Kitzinger, J. (1994). The methodology of focus groups: The importance of interaction between research participants, *Sociology of Health, 16*(1),136–142.

MacArthur, J., Kelly, B., and Higgins, N. (2005). Supporting the learning and social experiences of students with disabilities: What does the research say? In D. Fraser, R Moltzen, and K. Ryba (Eds.), *Learners with special needs in Aotearoa New Zealand* (pp. 49–73). Palmerston North, New Zealand: Thomson Press.

Mc Cracken, G. (1998). *The long interview: Qualitative Research Methods 13.* London: Sage.

Mayer, R. E. (2001). *Multimedia learning.* Cambridge, UK: Cambridge University Press.

Merton, R. K., and Kendall, P. L. (1946). The focused interview. *American Journal of Sociology,* 51, 541–557.

Meyer, L., and Bevan-Brown, J. (2005). Collaboration for social inclusion. In D. Fraser, R Moltzen, and K. Ryba (Eds.), *Learners with special needs in Aotearoa New Zealand* (pp. 168–192). Palmerston North, New Zealand: Thomson Press.

Minister for Disability Issues. (2001). *The New Zealand Disability Strategy: Making a world of difference Whakakauni Oranga.* Wellington: Ministry of Health.

Ministry of Education. (2004). *Enhancing effective practice in special education: A pilot study (research report)* Wellington, New Zealand: Author.

Ministry of Education. (2007). *National administration guidelines.* Wellington, New Zealand: Author.

Ministry of Health. (2001). *The New Zealand Disability Strategy: Making a world of difference Whakakauni Oranga. Pictorial Version.* Wellington, New Zealand: Author.

Morgan, D., and Krueger, R. (1993). When to use focus groups and why. In D. Morgan (Ed.), *Successful focus groups: Advancing the state of the art* (pp. 3–20). Newbury Park, CA: Sage.

Nakken, H., and Pijl, S. (2002). Getting along with classmates in regular schools—A review of the effects of integration on the development of social relationships. *International Journal of Inclusive Education, 6*(1), pp.47–61.

Sibbett, D. (1981). *I see what you mean: An introduction to graphic language recording and facilitation.* San Francisco: Sibbett and Associates.

Slee, R. (2001). Inclusion in practice: Does practice make perfect? *Educational Review, 53*(2), pp. 41–61.

Tierney, P. (2003). The competitive advantage of rich media. *American Bar Association (ABA) Journal,* 89(6), p. S4.

Waldegrave, C. (2003.).Focus groups. In C. Davidson, and M. Tolich (Eds.). *Social Science Research in New Zealand* (2nd ed.).(pp. 251–262) Auckland, New Zealand: Pearson.

Woolsey, K. (1996). *Vizability.* Boston: PWS Publishing Company.

AUTHOR NOTE

Deborah Espiner is a Principal Lecturer in the Faculty of Education, University of Auckland, New Zealand. She has a strong background in supporting students with disabilities within the education system. Deborah's considerable experience includes designing and teaching programmes for teachers and human service workers and facilitating Ministry of Education research contracts.

Diane Guild is the Manager of Professional Development and Outreach Services for Mt Richmond Special School, Auckland. Diane's experience includes teaching in all sectors and co-ordinating and facilitating Ministry of Education professional development and research contracts. She is committed to inclusion and the development of learning communities in school contexts.

The authors would like to thank the group of young people whose voices were the basis of this project. Without their energy, ideas, co-operation, and trust this chapter would not have been possible.

In: New Research in Education Adult, Medical and Vocational ISBN 978-1-60741-873-3
Editors: Edmondo Balistrieri and Giustino DeNino © 2009 Nova Science Publishers, Inc.

Chapter 7

STUDY GUIDES

M.H. Davis and G.G. Ponnamperuma
University of Dundee, Scotland, UK

ABSTRACT

Learner study guides are increasingly used in health professions' curricula. Their importance lies in their explicitness about what is to be taught and learned and their ability to identify the core. They are a key tool in the promotion of self-directed learning and tell the learners what to learn; how to learn it; and whether they have learned it.

Study guides have three roles: provision of content; management of learning; and student activities. Two models for study guide development are provided: TOPICAL for clinical courses; and TRACKER for distance learning. Convenience, language and readability, instructional design, and format need consideration when preparing a study guide.

The advantages of study guides include the ability to support the educational strategies of the institution and making education more effective. Potential disadvantages include: being too prescriptive and 'spoon-feeding'; queries about suitability for all learning styles; the teacher time involved in the development; being resource intensive; and the need for regular updating. These disadvantages, however, can be overcome in practice and are out weighed by the advantages. A model for the key features of study guides "the ten Is" is presented.

INTRODUCTION

"A study guide is an aid, usually presented in the form of printed notes or electronically produced, designed to facilitate studies" (Laidlaw and Hesketh, 2005). Study guides have been described as tutorials in print by Rowntree (1986), who is credited with their first use at the Open University in the UK. Study guides are used for both staff and students. Staff or tutor guides are sometimes used in problem-based curricula, to brief facilitators who may not be familiar with the content area of the problem-based learning session, or in other situations where it is necessary to brief staff about a teaching session or a course of study, such as trainers in out reach sites or peripheral hospitals. This article, however, will focus on student or learner study guides and it will be of interest to those wishing to evaluate the use of study guides for their own teaching and learn how to write and produce them. The article describes the importance of study guides and their role in the curriculum; provides models for study guide development and instructions for their preparation; and identifies the advantages and disadvantages of study guide use.

IMPORTANCE OF STUDY GUIDES

Study guides tell the learner what to learn, how to learn it and whether they have learned it (Harden et al., 1999a). The study guide identifies what the student has to learn; for example, by citing pages and paragraphs in text books, although it is not itself a textbook. The study guide contains the syllabus or timetable of learning opportunities, but goes further than the syllabus by identifying the learning outcomes of each component of the syllabus. It also contains self-assessment material to enable the learner to identify whether or not learning has been satisfactorily achieved.

Study guides are used increasingly in undergraduate, postgraduate and continuing education, suggesting that teachers and trainers, learners and trainees, and health care professionals find them useful learning aids. There are several reasons for this. Study guides help the learner cope with the increasing problem of curriculum and information overload by being explicit about what it is that the learner is expected to study and learn. Learners no longer need to become swamped by irrelevant material as the study guide identifies what is relevant. Study guides are flexible in that they can be used in association with a range of educational approaches. They can support the educational strategy of the institution, such as problem-based learning (PBL); outcome-based education; work-place learning; or blended learning (a mix of e-learning and face-to-face activities). They can also be used to introduce newer educational strategies such as student-centred, problem-based or integrated learning.

The study guide plays an important role in helping the learner plan his or her own learning, which is useful at a time when teachers are seeking to customise their teaching for individuals or groups within a course or curriculum and to promote independent learning. In PBL, where facilitators are not available, the study guide can include a list of essential learning issues to ensure the students appropriately cover all the learning issues, even those that the group may have failed to identify. Material from different disciplines can be included in the study guide to help the student integrate their learning.

THE ROLE OF STUDY GUIDES

Study guides have three roles in facilitating learning as shown in figure 1.

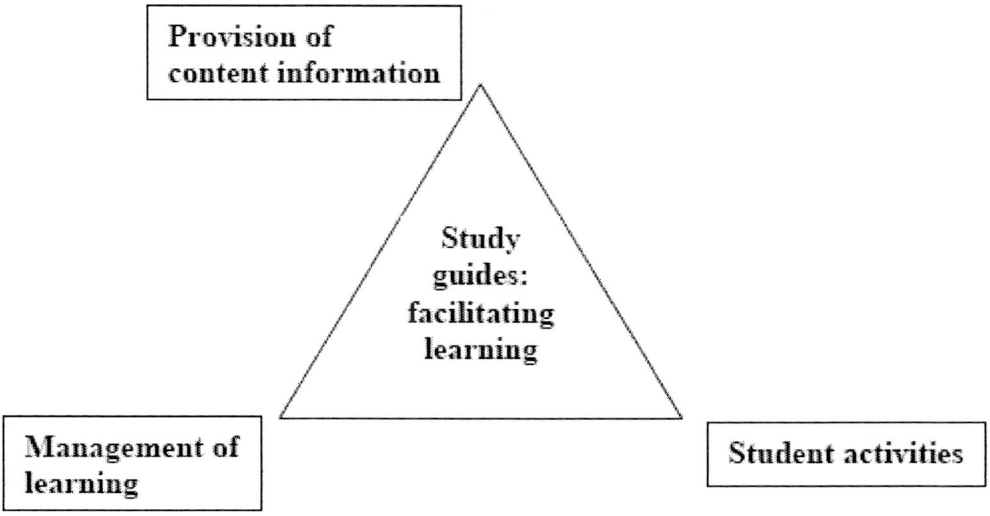

Figure1. The roles of a study guide.

A. Provision of Content Information

The important content that has to be learned is included in the study guide, preferably structured in terms of the learning outcomes of the course of study (Harden et al., 1999b). Thus the content material may include factual information and competencies that need to be mastered.

Factual information may be in the form of text (e.g. short notes, excerpts from books and journals) or graphics (e.g. diagrams, tables, photographs). This information could be either previously published information or new information. *Previously published information* may include: reference lists of textbooks and journals that constitute essential or further reading; quotations highlighting the main take-home messages; longer extracts (e.g. a paragraph or two) from the literature to reinforce the core concepts; and complete texts/articles if they are fundamentally important and short enough to go into a study guide. *New information* comprises: short notes or comments on the topic by the tutor; core-information; a more extended account of an important aspect of the topic; and a glossary of keywords or technical terms. The latter is particularly important if PBL is a major learning strategy of the course, as failure to understand jargon is one of the factors that impedes learning in PBL. In general, the new information that the authors decide to include in the study guide should either supplement or/and complement what is already available to the learners or address particular aspects that the teachers wish to emphasise. The temptation to overload the study guide with information needs to be avoided, as this may defeat the very reason for introducing a study guide; i.e. to focus the learners on the main learning points.

Arranging the above information within a framework such as the *outcomes* or *competencies* that the learners need to master will give direction to both the learners and teachers. In a recent study, however, by Khogali et al. (2006) that compared three study guide frameworks (i.e. outcome-based, timetable-based, and problem-based), the second-year medical students of Dundee Medical School, Scotland, UK preferred the timetable-based, study-guide framework.

B. Assistance in the Management of Learning

Provision of a menu of learning opportunities is an important role for the study guide. Different learners may prefer different learning styles and approaches: independent study; group work; learning by doing; on-line learning; discussions with tutors; clinical skills sessions and so on. If the study guide identifies the available learning opportunities, the learner can plan his or her learning making use of the educational opportunities that match his or her needs and preferred ways of learning.

Provision of the following material facilitates the learners' management of their own learning: overview of the topic (i.e. what the learners should expect during the course); pre-requisites (what the learners should know before starting the course); timetable (at what point will different topics be introduced during the course); learning outcomes (what the learners should achieve at the end of the course); learning strategies (approach to teaching and learning; e.g. PBL, community-based learning); learning opportunities (the teaching sessions provided for the learners by the institution; e.g. seminars; lectures; project work; clinical skills sessions); the resources available for independent study (e.g. relevant books in the library with specific pages identified for study; websites and how to access them; and computer assisted learning material); assessment (how the achievement of learning outcomes will be checked during and/or at the end of the course); staff contact details (how learners can clarify queries); and personal comments by authors (what the authors need to stress, the key steps to the successful completion of the course, and any pitfalls to avoid during the course).

C. Provision of Activities

Activities are included in the study guide to help learners interact with the material they have to learn, in order to internalise their learning. The activities may include questions to answer, tasks to undertake, self-assessment exercises and aspects on which the learner should reflect – "think points". For example, in a study guide on 'outcome-based education' once the learners have been introduced to the disadvantages of 'outcome-based education', an appropriate think point may be:

Do you see these as disadvantages in your setting/institution? How might these be overcome?

The activities that can be built into the study guide may help learners: understand new learning based on what is already known (i.e. schema building); reinforce what has been taught (e.g. prescribing activities after each learning session); link different learning experiences (i.e. integrating theory with practice, integrating learning from different disciplines and topics); check whether learning has been achieved (e.g. self-assessment); and record achievement of learning outcomes. These records may be used as portfolio items. The record of activities may contribute to a personal information bank on the subject. The advent of e-learning has focused attention on the development of a learner's personal information bank. In some American medical schools learner handouts are given as a hypertext programme guide so that the learner can cross-reference and inter-relate different pieces of information introduced during the course (Laidlaw and Harden, 1990). In short, the learner activities in the study guide should facilitate 'deep learning'. Learner feedback is another important activity that can be incorporated into a study guide. A 'feedback form', with a perforated tear-off line or able to be submitted electronically, included at the end of the study guide will enable the course designers to improve the guide as well as the course in the future.

The balance between the three roles varies in individual study guides, giving great variation in format. Some study guides may focus mainly on provision of content information, some on the management of learning, while others mainly provide student activities. Many study guides, however, fulfil all three roles.

The study guide contributes to a supportive, student-centred educational environment (Roff and McAleer, 2001) providing the overarching ambience, within which directed learning takes place.

WHAT GOES INTO A STUDY GUIDE: MODELS FOR STUDY GUIDE DEVELOPMENT

The content of a study guide can be described using two mnemonics or models: TOPICAL (Mires et al., 1998) and TRACKER (Laidlaw, 2005).

T opics	**T** argets
O bjectives	**R** oute of study
P rogramme of work	**A** ssessment acitivities
I ssues for learning	**C** ore information
C linical tasks	**K** ey tips
A ssessment	**E** ducational opportunities
L og book	**R** eadable material

Figure 2. Two models for the content of a study guide.

Topical

Topics provide a summary list of the material with which the course deals. *Objectives* are what the learner should achieve at the end of the course; i.e. course-level outcomes. These objectives can be linked to the overall exit learning outcomes of the institute so that both the students and teachers know how each course contributes to the achievement of the overall aims and outcomes of the institution. The Scottish Dental Vocational Guide (Harden et al., 1989) provides a list of tasks and shows how each relates to the learning outcomes. The *programme of work* details how the learner should set about tackling a topic and sequence his/her work. It includes a reference list where the learners can obtain further information on the topic. Details of relevant clinics, wards or theatre, where clinical material related to the topic can be found may also be provided. As the programme of work directs the learner to the relevant reading as well as relevant clinical material, it provides the critical link between theory and practice. *Issues for learning* may be a series of questions with answers provided at the end of the study guide. This provides material for the learner to self-assess their knowledge. The study guide may also prescribe *clinical tasks*. On completion of these tasks the learners are required to document them in a *log book*. Later, the logbook entries can be submitted for *assessment* marked by the tutor and returned to the student with feedback. For example, the study guide may suggest that the learner should take clinical histories and perform physical examination on patients with specific disorders. The learner records the history and examination findings in a log book. At the end of the rotation the learner submits the logbook for assessment (Mires et al., 1998) by the tutor. The logbook is then returned to the student with feedback regarding aspects of clinical competence, such as history taking, physical examination, and patient investigations and management.

As opposed to the strong clinical orientation of TOPICAL, the TRACKER model has a more generic structure and has been used extensively in distance learning.

Tracker

Targets are synonymous with course outcomes or objectives. *Route of study* prescribes the sequence of learning activities that the learner should follow to achieve the targets. It is similar to the 'programme of work' of the TOPICAL model. *Assessment* covers self and external assessment, both formative and summative. *Core information* refers to the essential course material that the students have to master; i.e. the 'core-curriculum'. It also provides information on where to find relevant and important material. *Key tips* can be used to highlight important aspects of the topic, provide advice based on practical experience or put the area of study into context. The following is a key tip from a study guide for junior doctors working in paediatrics in Scotland (Mitchell, 1996).

If this is your first paediatric SHO post you will probably feel quite nervous at the prospect of being on call and dealing with emergencies. The senior staff will expect and recognise this.

They are the 'words of wisdom' passed from the tutor to the learner. Key tips may link theory to practice as they can provide important practical aids when applying the course material to clinical/practical situations. For example, a study guide on the OSCE (Objective Structured Clinical Examination) contains the following key tip.

The reliability of exam results is linked to the length of testing time. Use as many stations as feasible in an OSCE. Research has shown approximately 18-25 stations are needed to provide reliable results.

The first sentence of the above passage provides the *theory* or the principle. The other sentences then link this principle to *practice* by advising on the optimal number of OSCE stations for an OSCE. All the above features of key tips facilitate active and deep learning.

Educational opportunities refers to the various learning resources and activities available to the learners; e.g. lectures; textbooks; small group activities; clinical tasks; seminars; library resources or websites. *Readable material* suggests that the content of the study guide should be an easy read or user-friendly for the learners, written in a style and at a level that the target audience can understand. This contributes to a supportive learner-centred educational environment.

As shown in table 1, both TOPICAL and TRACKER contain similar content.

Table 1. A comparison of the content in two study guide structures: TOPICAL and TRACKER

Aspect addressed by the study guide	TOPICAL	TRACKER
What the learner should be able to do at the end of the course.	O bjectives	T argets
Content that the learner should learn.	T opics	C ore information
How the learners may learn.	P rogramme of work	R oute of study
How the learner can know that (s)he has learned.	I ssues for learning - Assessment	A ssessment activities
Aids for reflection or application of learning.	C linical tasks – Logbook – Assessment	K ey tips
Learning resources.	P rogramme of work C linical tasks – Logbook	R oute of study R eadable material E ducational opportunities

Blending the models TOPICAL and TRACKER forms TOP CARE (figure 3) – the educational 'care' that the course developer can provide for the learner through a study guide.

T ips – key tips; think points
O bjectives / targets
P rogramme of work / route of study

C ore information / topics
A ssessment / issues for learning
R esources for learning / educational opportunities
E ducational environment

Figure 3.'Top care' from a study guide for the learner: the content of a study guide.

INSTRUCTIONS FOR STUDY GUIDE PREPARATION

Several practical issues need to be addressed in the preparation of a study guide. Careful attention to these practical issues can make the difference between a well used study guide and one that is ignored.

Convenience

The guide must be convenient to use when and where the learner wishes to use it. For print-based study guides, attention needs to be paid to the size of the guide. Does it, for example, need to fit into the pocket of a white coat? Would lamination of the pages increase its usable life? Alternatively, should the study guide be provided electronically? If it is sufficiently large does it need to be divided into sections?

Language and Readability

Readability is essential and the guide has to be pitched at a level the readers will understand. Familiar words rather than esoteric language aid understanding and readability. The FOGG index (Owen, 2008) provides a measure to evaluate the readability. Short simple sentences and the active rather than the passive voice tend to make information more readily understood.

Instructional Design

The use of *advance organisers* will prepare learners for new experiences. An advance organiser may take the form of a list of headings that will be worked through or an overview at the top of the page indicating what the page is about. *Headings* are important for indicating to the learner what the section is about and also for disciplining the writer to structure the content. Headings make the information easier for the learner to assimilate. *Illustrations* such as photographs, graphs, charts or cartoons, are useful if they support learning; for example, by demonstrating something that would take many words to describe; illustrating a complex concept or helping the learner to remember key points. Cartoons can be helpful for the same purpose but care has to be taken to use them to lighten the mood without trivialising the content. Cartoons can add humour and keep the learner's attention. Humour, however, has to be used with care and without causing offence. Illustrations and cartoons should never be used without a learning purpose. In such circumstances they act as distractors and open the writer to criticism.

Format

With print-based study guides, consideration has to be given to the number of copies required. It is usually cost effective to use a commercial printing company if hundreds of copies are required but the disadvantage is that, once printed, the material cannot readily be changed or updated. A more professional appearance is usually achieved with commercially printed material but the flexibility of in-house production with a word-processing package may be desirable where regular updates of the study guide are necessary for each cohort of learners. The costs of commercial printing are an added expense for the institution and it may be difficult or inappropriate in some institutions to pass on the costs to the learners. Electronic distribution can seem to be an easy option for the institution, but often results in learners printing out the guide thus passing on the printing costs from the institution to the learners. This may be inappropriate in an age when health professions' learners graduate with large debts.

The use of colour is beguiling as the study guide looks more attractive but it will add to the cost and should only be used if educationally essential; for example, to indicate different sections for ease of use, or if high quality colour photographs are essential for understanding the content.

The type of paper used for the guide is another consideration, both in terms of weight (thickness) and finish. Thicker paper adds to the overall quality of the guide and is essential if the guide is to be printed on both sides of the paper, but it is more expensive and heavier to carry or post in the mail than thinner alternatives. Thinner paper is less opaque and print may be seen through the page, acting as a distractor and reducing readability. If the paper is too thin, it can only be printed on one side, which may potentially double the weight of the guide and increase costs such as printing, mailing and distribution. Matt paper can look highly professional. Glossy paper looks attractive but it can be difficult to write annotations on and to read in artificial light because of glare.

Communication on-line, as in electronic study guides, is a burgeoning industry. As experience grows rules and principles are developing. Electronic study guides are increasingly used and Montemayor (2002) has provided guidelines for their preparation. It is likely, however, that this will be a fast changing field for some time to come.

Advantages of Study Guides

Study guides assist learning by making it convenient, relevant, interesting, systematic, individualised, amenable to self-assessment, and speculative; i.e. study guides support the CRISIS model of effective education (Harden and Laidlaw, 1992). Study guides are *convenient* as they can be used for quick guidance in learning situations where reference to standard textbooks may not be possible; e.g. during a busy clinic or in the operating theatre. They are *relevant* as the study guide is designed specifically for the individual course of study. Learners' *interest* in the subject may be aroused by the user-friendly presentation of the content in a study guide, and the use of icons and graphics, etc. Paying attention to the layout of the study guide also adds interest. Study guides direct the learner through the learning material in a logical, step-wise sequence and identify all the core content to be learned. They are thus *systematic*. Study guides help the learner plan an *individualised* learning programme, depending on the learner needs. Most study guides have *self-assessment* questions for the learner to verify whether he/she has mastered the content. Study guides can also indicate any controversial or 'grey' areas in the subject e.g., dubiety about the definitive treatment for a specified condition, and thus expose areas open for *speculation,* debate or further research.

DISADVANTAGES OF STUDY GUIDES

There are fears, however, that study guides:

- may place restrictions on learning. This may de-motivate the more enthusiastic learner. Identifying the core that all the learners should achieve, however, is not a restriction on the more capable learners. The study guide identifies the basic minimum that all learners should achieve, but can also direct the more able learner to more advanced learning material clearly identified as such.
- encourage 'spoon-feeding' and thus may not prepare the learners for life-long learning. On the contrary, the study guide encourages the learners to take responsibility for their own learning and hence prepares learners for life-long learning.
- may not be suitable for certain learning styles. Study guides, however, can identify for the learner a wide range of learning opportunities, so that the learner can choose what best suits her/him.
- require considerable teacher time, skill and experience to design. This is true, but any good course requires teacher time, expertise and experience. Once produced, annual updates of study guides are not time consuming to achieve.
- require substantial physical resources; e.g. stationery, printing, computers. Study guide production can indeed be costly and there are issues as to who bears the cost; e.g. the institution or the learner.
- need regular updating to reflect the current research findings and trends. This is part of good teaching. Any teaching material needs updating to prevent it becoming obsolete.
- may discourage learners to refer to more authoritative textbooks. If, however, the material included in the study guide is judiciously chosen, the references in the study guide could encourage learners to refer to more advanced material such as specialised publications/articles, where appropriate.
- may threaten learner autonomy. The propagators of 'education for its own sake' and 'discovery learning' criticise study guides as being too 'prescriptive'. It can be argued, however, that avoidance of information overload necessitates prescriptive definition of the core. On the other hand, study guides train learners to manage their own learning and thus encourage autonomous, independent learning.
- are difficult to update once printed. If, however, study guides are available in electronic format or in a printed 'Word' version, they are easily updated.

SUMMARY

The key features of study guides can be summarised as 10 I s (Davis and Harden, 2000). Study guides are:

1. Important, in terms of contributions they can make to the education process.
2. Interesting for the learner, if appropriately designed.
3. Immediately available for the learner.
4. Inspiring or motivating for the learner.
5. Informative in communicating to learners and teachers what the learner needs to know.
6. Illustrative, by illustrating theory with practical examples.
7. Integrating, by bringing together different disciplines, different contexts for learning such as the hospital and community, and linking theory to practice.
8. Interactive, with active involvement of the learner.
9. Iterative, encouraging the learner to revisit areas previously studied and to build on their knowledge or an understanding of the topic.
10. Impacting, with potentially a profound effect on the learner.

REFERENCES

Davis, M.H., and Harden, R.M. (2000). Study guides. No. 8, in: *Good ideas about medical education*. Dundee, UK: Centre for Medical Education, University of Dundee, p2.

Harden, R., Crosby, J., and Davis, M.H. (1999b). An introduction to outcome-based education. *Medical Teacher* 21:7-14.

Harden, R.M., and Laidlaw, J.M. (1992). Effective continuing education: the CRISIS criteria. *Medical Education* 26:408-256.

Harden, R.M., Laidlaw, J.M., and Hesketh, E.A. (1999a). AMEE Guide No 16: Study guides: their use and preparation. *Medical Teacher* 21:248-265.

Harden, R.M., Laidlaw, J.M., Abdel-Fattah, A.M.A., Dryden, J.M., Nicoll, G.O., Robb, I.M., and Steed, M.S. (1989). *Training Guide – Scottish Dental Vocational Training Committee.* Dundee, UK: Centre for Medical Education, University of Dundee.

Khogali, S.E., Laidlaw, J.M., and Harden, R.M. (2006). Study guides: a study of different formats. *Medical Teacher* 28:375-377.

Laidlaw, J., and Hesketh, E. (2005). Study guides. In: Dent JA, Harden RM. (Eds.) *A practical guide for medical teachers.* Edinburgh, UK: Elsevier Churchill Livingston, p194-200.

Laidlaw, J.M. (2005). *Study guides: Instructional Material Design (IMD) Unit 9.* Dundee, UK: Centre for Medical Education, University of Dundee, p1.

Laidlaw, J.M., and Harden, R.M. (1990). What is.........a study guide? *Medical Teacher* 12:7-12.

Mires, G.J., Howie, P.W., and Harden, R.M. (1998). A 'topical' approach to planned teaching learning using a topic-based study guide. *Medical Teacher* 20:438-441.

Mitchell, H. (1996). *Learning Paediatrics – A Training Guide for Senior House Officers.* Dundee, UK: Centre for Medical Education, University of Dundee.

Montemayor, L. (2002). Twelve tips for the development of electronic study guides. *Medical Teacher* 24:473-478.

Owen, A. (2008). *Readability: beyond the basics.* (2008 December 21). Available from: http://www.writershelper.com/readability.html.

Roff, S., and McAleer, S. (2001). What is educational climate? *Medical Teacher* 23(4):333-334.

Rowntree, D. (1986). *Teaching through self-instruction.* London, UK: Kogan Page, p91.

This work supported in part by unrestricted grant from Research to Prevent Blindness, Inc., N.Y., N.Y.

In: New Research in Education Adult, Medical and Vocational ISBN 978-1-60741-873-3
Editors: Edmondo Balistrieri and Giustino DeNino © 2009 Nova Science Publishers, Inc.

Chapter 8

The Impact of the New ACGME Competencies on Graduate Medical Education: The Ophthalmology Experience

Andrew G. Lee[1]
Departments of Ophthalmology, Neurology, and Neurosurgery (AGL) at the H. Stanley Thompson Neuro-ophthalmology Clinic, the University of Iowa Hospitals and Clinics, IA, USA

Abstract

The apprenticeship model for teaching tha art and science medicine has long been the mainstay of graduate medical education (GME). Significant change in the health care environment however has resulted in a new set of challenges and growing public and private calls for reform in the GME process. In response to these calls, there has been an emerging consensus to move from the traditional "apprenticeship model" to a new "competency model" of education. External and internal stakeholders in the health care system (e.g., regulatory agencies, private nongovernmental professional organizations, insurance companies, industry, and the public) now demand "proof of quality" based upon evidence, external measures of performance, data driven improvements, and quantifiable outcomes. Due in part to these external pressures new competencies have emerged for GME that will require the development of new tools to both teach and assess "competence" in the "competencies". The Accreditation Council for Graduate Medical Education (ACGME) in the United States has proposed six specific new competencies including patient care, medical knowledge, communication and interpersonal skills, professionalism, practice based learning, and systems based practice.

This short communication will describe the six ACGME competencies, the emerging tools that might be used to both teach and assess these competencies; the current concepts and educational models guiding tool development and testing, and the results of an implementation process in the field of ophthalmology. The new ACGME competencies will require the development and testing of specific tools that will form the basis of a

[1] Address correspondence to Andrew G. Lee, MD, Department of Ophthalmology, 200 Hawkins Dr. PFP, University of Iowa Hospitals and Clinics, Iowa City, IA 52242, 319-384-7372, 319-353-7996 (fax), andrew-lee@uiowa.edu.

competency toolbox. These tools ideally would include both formative and summative feedback, faculty oversight, structured learning activities, specific scoring rubrics with behavioral anchors, benchmark and aggregate data, and linkage to improved downstream patient outcomes (e.g., quality, medical error reduction, patient safety, cost effectiveness). The barriers to implementation as well as examples of small successes and progress will be described. The challenge for organized medicine is developing an integrated, systematic, reliable and valid approach for GME to move from the "apprenticeship model" towards a "competency based" model.

INTRODUCTION

The traditional "apprenticeship model" (learning by observing and training with an experienced mentor) has been at the core of graduate medical education (GME) in the United States since before the days of Osler. Unfortunately external pressures have emerged that have prompted calls for reforming the GME process and one proposed solution has been to create a new competency based model. This short communication will include he following: 1) To list the six Accrediation Council for Graduate Medical Education (ACGME) competencies; 2) To define the emerging tools that might be used to both teach and assess these competencies; 3) To discuss the current concepts and educational models guiding teaching tool development and testing, and 4) To describe the results of an implementation process using the author's GME experience in the specialty of ophthalmology.

The ACGME embarked on a comprehensive and inclusive process to define six specific competencies for graduate medical education. The process involved multiple internal and external stakeholders, a literature review, a consensus building process, and an iterative reduction of principles that was consolidated into the new competencies. Table 1 lists the six ACGME competencies (www.acgme.org).

Table 1. The ACGME competencies (from www.ACGME.org)

a) *Patient Care t*hat is compassionate, appropriate, and effective for the treatment of health problems and the promotion of health
b) *Medical Knowledge* about established and evolving biomedical, clinical, and cognate (e.g. epidemiological and social-behavioral) sciences and the application of this knowledge to patient care
c) *Practice-Based Learning and Improvement* that involves investigation and evaluation of their own patient care, appraisal and assimilation of scientific evidence, and improvements in patient care
d) *Interpersonal and Communication Skills* that result in effective information exchange and teaming with patients, their families, and other health professionals
e) *Professionalism,* as manifested through a commitment to carrying out professional responsibilities, adherence to ethical principles, and sensitivity to a diverse patient population
f) *Systems-Based Practice*, as manifested by actions that demonstrate an awareness of and responsiveness to the larger context and system of health care and the ability to effectively call on system resources to provide care that is of optimal value

After finalizing the six competencies, the ACGME defined a 10-year "Outcome project". This Outcome Project is an ambitious and national mandate to improve GME through the teaching and assessing of the six competencies across all medical residents (see Table 1). The ACGME has defined the following goals for the "Outcome Project" : 1) To identify learning objectives related to the ACGME general competencies; 2) To use increasingly more dependable, objective methods of assessing resident attainment of competency-based objectives; and 3) To use outcome data to facilitate continuous improvement of both individual resident and residency programmatic performance. The strategies for the Outcome Project to achieve these goals are listed below.[1]

1. "Development of a set of general competencies;
2. Support for programs through identification and development of dependable methods for assessing attainment of the competencies;
3. Development of model resident evaluation systems to provide examples of dependable evaluation; and,
4. Creation of a support system of resources that includes assessment experts, ideas for teaching the general competencies, references for articles pertinent to the definition, teaching and evaluation of the competencies, and a "toolbox" of assessment techniques"[1]

Over the course of the first several phases of the project, the ACGME initially relied upon educational innovation from program directors and like minded educators to build selected tools. Over the course of time tools have emerged that may be suitable for specific individual or multiple competencies. Table 2 lists the available tools in the toolbox.

Table 2. Selected tools in the ACGME "toolbox" (from the www.ACGME.org)

1. Direct observation concurrent evaluation and other focused assessment methods
2. Multi-source or 360-degree evaluations (e.g., peers, patients, staff, students, self and other non-MD members of the care team)
3. Structured checklist evaluations, self reflection exercises and self improvement projects with documentation in a learning portfolio
4. Cognitive oral and written tests

Despite the consensus regarding the need for implantation of the "toolbox", the ACGME Outcomes Project, remains essentially an unfunded mandate at the local level. In addition, the precise logistical details were not provided to the medical and surgical specialties and the practical implementation issues were left to the specialties and individual institutions and GME programs themselves.[2-4]

We previously outlined our academic institution's (The University of Iowa Hospital and Clinics Department of Ophthalmology) implementation plan2; summarized the existing GME literature; gleaned selected best practices from the review; and reviewed the existing tools in the ACGME assessment "tool box".[2-14] Tables 3 and 4 summarize the major aspects of our implementation program.

Table 3. The University of Iowa Department of Ophthalmology Implementation Plan for Managing the ACGME Outcomes Project

1. Form an intramural Task Force devoted to the competencies. At the University of Iowa's Department of Ophthalmology we formalized our competency assessment process by creating an ad hoc Departmental Task Force on the Competencies. The purpose of the Task Force was to create a cadre of "like-minded" individuals, to divide the labor, and to develop a multi-pronged approach to implement multiple tools from the 'toolbox" in the shortest period of time. The Iowa Task Force was composed of faculty members who volunteered to participate, the program director (who served as the Task Force chair), the fellowship program director, the medical student director, and the chair of the Department.
2. Review the mission. An ongoing review of the mission, goals, and objectives of the Task Force was performed each year in order to define the specific cultural, institutional, and resource barriers to full compliance with the ACGME mandate.
3. Use multiple tools. We use multiple tools over multiple encounters, with multiple assessors to assess the individual specific and overlapping competencies.
4. Use tools that are reliable, valid, and feasible. The Task Force defined face and content validity for the selected tools and deployed methods to improve reliability (training raters, using defined scoring rubrics, and providing forums for public discussion about tool design, strengths, and weaknesses.
5. Ask less work from more people. Division of labor and spreading the workload across the Department was used to minimize faculty burden and time commitment but also to create pride of ownership, to foster a culture of competency, and to increase public visibility of the process.
6. Develop quantitative data-driven external (to the program) and internal programmatic outcome measures. In Phase 3 of the ACGME Outcome Project there will be a clear demand for measures of programmatic and individual improvement and success that are derived from outside of the Department (i.e., external outcome measures).
7. Insure fairness. Transparency and accountability were keys to the initial buy in" and continued sustainability for the process. This includes defining explicit, written and publicly available learning objectives in a structured educational curriculum for both teachers and learners.
8. Use formative feedback. Formative feedback is the basis of our programmatic efforts to improve performance by providing timely, specific, and behavior related feedback that can then be used to create a rich, multidimensional profile for summative feedback (i.e., the "final grade").
9. Use the results. All results of the assessment process are used to motivate individual and programmatic improvement over time
10. Define learner and programmatic benchmarks. We advocate for the creation of a national database of aggregate and individual programmatic but redacted (i.e., anonymous and confidential) data that can be used for benchmarking purposes and to define linkage to downstream outcome improvements in the quality of patient care, reduction of medical error, improved cost effectiveness, or increased efficiency in delivery of care.

Table 4. Tools implemented at the University of Iowa Department of Ophthalmology

1. The University of Iowa ophthalmology residency curriculum (based in part upon a modified version of the International Council of Ophthalmology (ICO) curriculum for residents and specialists). The ICO curriculum has been recognized as an ACGME "good practice" (www.acgme.org)
2. Direct observation using the Ophthalmic Clinical Exercise (OCEX)
3. Journal club tool using a structured format and review checklist
4. Multi-source evaluation tool (i.e, the 360 degree evaluation)
5. A modified Dreyfus scale faculty global evaluation form
6. The Iowa Cataract Surgical Curriculum using formative structured objective assessments of technical skill (modified OSATS) and incorporates deliberate practice
7. The Iowa Ophthalmic Laser curriculum
8. The Iowa Ophthalmic Wet Lab (OWL) curriculum
9. Traditional written and oral examinations for medical knowledge
10. Self reflection exercises and projects presented at ophthalmology grand rounds and then published on line (www.eyerounds.org)
11. Learner portfolio that includes demographic information, test results, evaluation forms, and all of the results of the above evaluations.

SUMMARY

The ACGME Outcome Project is a multiyear, ambitious, important, "sea-change" in GME. Although much progress has been made, it is my opinion that the ACGME process is at a critical "tipping point". The GME reform process could collapse from any number of external and internal threats including apathy, competency "fatigue", disengagement by the specialties, institutional, specialty, or organization backlash, or even an outright "mutiny". Alternatively the process can continue to grow and flourish and ultimately achieve the original aspirational goals for improving not just GME but also the quality, satisfaction, cost effectiveness, safety, and delivery of health care. The success of the project will require proof of direct linkage with defined improvements in downstream outcomes (e.g., patient satisfaction, quality of care improvement, cost savings, improved efficiency and reduction of medical errors). This quantitative external "hard data" will be necessary to squelch the growing body of "nay-sayers" to the process.

Educational innovation and reform requires some risk, specific tools need to be developed and tested in the real world and novel revenue streams will need to be diverted to the effort as the ACGME mandate remains unfunded. Programs participating in the educational experimentation need to have incentives (e.g., extended review cycles, public recognition of "best practices", outlets for academic promotion and scholarly activity) to continue to divert precious clinical, research, and faculty resources towards GME.

Invigoration of the process, creation of momentum and sustainability mechanisms, and proof of efficacy will be needed in the next few years to reverse faculty and programmatic "competency fatigue", apathy, and any potential "backlash".

Although local implementation at the "grass roots" level at places like the University of Iowa has demonstrated modest success, national engagement by all of the organizational, accrediting, and credentialing stakeholders, cross-organizational "buy in", and standardized implementation mechanisms will be necessary to insure long term success.

References

[1] Accreditation Council for Graduate Medical Education website http://www.acgme.org/outcome/about/faq.asp (last accessed July 12, 2008).

[2] Lee AG, Carter KD. Managing the new mandate in resident education: a blueprint for translating a national mandate into local compliance. Ophthalmology 2004;111:1807-12.

[3] Lee AG, Volpe N. The impact of the new competencies on resident education in ophthalmology. Ophthalmology 2004;111:1269-70.

[4] Lee AG. The new competencies and their impact on resident training in ophthalmology. Surv Ophthalmol 2003;48:651-62.

[5] Lee AG, Beaver HA, Greenlee E, et al. Teaching and assessing systems-based competency in ophthalmology residency training programs. Surv Ophthalmol 2007;52:680-9.

[6] Lee AG, Beaver HA, Boldt HC, et al. Teaching and assessing professionalism in ophthalmology residency training programs. Surv Ophthalmol 2007;52:300-14.

[7] Oetting TA, Lee AG, Beaver HA, et al. Teaching and assessing surgical competency in ophthalmology training programs. Ophthalmic Surg Lasers Imaging 2006;37:384-93.

[8] Lee AG, Boldt HC, Golnik KC, et al. Using the Journal Club to teach and assess competence in practice-based learning and improvement: a literature review and recommendation for implementation. Surv Ophthalmol 2005;50:542-8.

[9] Golnik KC, Lee AG, Carter K. Assessment of ophthalmology resident on-call performance. Ophthalmology 2005;112:1242-6.

[10] Lee AG and Carter K. OCEX Reliability. Ophthalmology 2007; 113: 717 – 717.

[11] Golnik KC, Goldenhar L. The ophthalmic clinical evaluation exercise: reliability determination. Ophthalmology 2005;112:1649-54.

[12] Golnik KC, Goldenhar LM, Gittinger JW Jr, Lustbader JM. The Ophthalmic Clinical Evaluation Exercise (OCEX). Ophthalmology 2004;111:1271-4.

[13] Oetting TA, Beaver HA, Johnson AT, et al. Planning for Surgical Competency: The University of Iowa experience (in press, J Acad Ophthalmology).

[14] Graff J, Oetting TA, Lee AG. The Ophthalmic Knowledge Assessment Program (OKAP) Examination and Global Evaluation of Resident Performance. J Acad Ophthalmology 2008;1:20-24.

Table 5. Outlines the University of Iowa Implementation Matrix for the ACGME competencies

Medical knowledge

What to Assess	How to Assess
Medical knowledge	Absolute and relative in service examination (i.e., OKAP) scores Pass rates on the American Board of Ophthalmology (ABO) written and oral qualifying exam Individual service oral examinations Global faculty evaluation

Patient care

What to Assess	How to Assess
Resident's overall patient care abilities in clinic	Global faculty performance rating Cataract surgery formative feedback forms using modified objective structured assessment of technical skills (OSATS) forms And 360° Assessment including technical staff, self assessments, patient satisfaction questionnaires
Clinical history and exam	Direct observation and evaluation of complete patient encounters with a structured scoring rubric and checklist (i.e., the Ophthalmic Clinical Exercise or OCEX)

Interpersonal and Communication Skills

What to Assess	How to Assess
Resident's overall interpersonal and communication skills during a rotation	Global faculty performance rating Observed consent for cataract surgery And 360° Assessment
Communication with outside physicians and patients by phone	Focused observation and evaluation using phone tool structured checklist

Professionalism

What to Assess	How to Assess
Ethics knowledge	Sentinel event (i.e., outstanding behavior or professional or ethics breaches or medical error or near miss) trigger self reflection exercise and face to face faculty discussion on impact of sentinel event Eyerounds.org case AND Praise or Criticism "cards" generated at time of sentinel event
Professional behaviors	360° Assessment with structured checklist of professional behaviors
The learning environment	Annual ACGME surveys, biannual anonymous electronic surveys (E-Value) and exit interview questionnaires completed by the residents

Practice-based Learning and Improvement

What to Assess	How to Assess
Processes and behaviors Reflection on practice and practice analysis Utilization of current literature A plan for change/improvement	Cataract Surgery Morbidity Conference Eyerounds.org case Portfolio with checklist assessment documenting presentations, publications, and journal club And Discussion-based assessment (e.g., chart stimulated recall) AND Global performance rating AND Journal Club tool (documentation of evidence based learning, written review for portfolio)
Outcomes, i.e., performance improvements	Presentation at grand rounds and reporting of case vignette on web site devoted to education (i.e., EyeRounds).
Portfolio	Written learning plan Evidence of self directed learning Time management diary including adherence to duty hour requirements Sentinel events documented Revised learning plan prompted by critical events

Systems based care

What to Assess	How to Assess
Systems based care: interaction of ophthalmology and health care system including other providers	Web based vignette and portfolio documentation Attendance at grand rounds presentations on SBL
2. Patient related systems based problem solving	Focused observation and faculty global evaluation On call chart audit for system errors and recommendations for system improvements Identification of system errors or improvements and publication of results in web based format (i.e., EyeRounds) Portfolio documentation of self reflection and system based repairs as appropriate

Surgery

What to Assess	How to Assess
Informed consent	Global performance rating AND Direct observation checklist
Identification of instruments	Web based tutorial Surgical curriculum Simulator and Wet lab curriculum pre and post testing Iowa retinal laser curriculum
Surgical skills: critical events	Cataract Morbidity Conference: Video review and critique with faculty surgeon of every intraoperative complication
Surgical technique	Direct observation checklist using global rating scale of operative performance (e.g., respect for tissue, time and motion, instrument handling, knowledge of instruments, flow of operation, use of assistants, knowledge of specific procedure)

In: New Research in Education Adult, Medical and Vocational ISBN 978-1-60741-873-3
Editors: Edmondo Balistrieri and Giustino DeNino © 2009 Nova Science Publishers, Inc.

Chapter 9

THEORY IN MEDICAL EDUCATION

David Kaufman
Faculty of Education,
Simon Fraser University, British Columbia

ABSTRACT

This chapter asserts that "there is nothing more practical than a good theory", and. as professional practice is better understood, theory will both inform practice and to be informed by it. Already, a body of theory has accumulated which can inform practice, and the author shows this by reviewing conclusions drawn from his earlier monograph on the application of eight educational theories to medical education. This is followed by a discussion of three different theories: cognitive apprenticeship, multiple intelligences, , and conditions of learning. A brief overview is provided of each of these theories followed by a discussion of their implications for educational practice., including a specific example for each drawn from medical education.

INTRODUCTION

Can educational theory inform our practice? Fortunately, the field of education, and medical education in particular, has come a long way in recent years. A body of theory has accumulated which can inform practice [1,2] However, there has been an unfortunate gap between academics and practitioners, which has led to a perception of theory as 'ivory tower' and not relevant to practice. Yet the old adage that "there is nothing more practical than a good theory" still rings true today, and. as professional practice is better understood, theory will both inform practice and to be informed by it.

My purpose in this exposition is to outline several selected educational theories, and to explore their implications for the practice of medical education. For the purposes of this paper, I use the term "theory" in a general sense, that is, as a set of assumptions and ideas that help to explain some phenomenon. Knowles addressed this topic more than 25 years ago, proposing a definition of a theory as, "a comprehensive, coherent, and internally consistent system of ideas about a set of phenomena." Each of the theoretical approaches that I describe here is consistent with Knowles' definition. Extensive research shows that we learn best through a combination of theory and practice [3]. Theory is inert until it is applied to a realistic situation, and practice is shallow without the influence of theory. A clear example is how modern surgeons are trained. Though learning the theory by attending lectures and reading books are necessary, this is not sufficient training for a surgeon. There is an obvious need for practical experience. In medical education, learners learn best by applying theory and techniques to realistic cases in either simulated environments where they can make mistakes without the serious consequences of failure, or in authentic settings where they can receive expert support.

In an earlier monograph, my colleague and I discussed eight theories: adult learning principles, social cognitive theory, reflective practice, transformative learning, self-directed learning, experiential learning, situated learning, and communities of practice [1]. In that publication, we outlined the following consistent messages that can be drawn from all of them to inform teaching and learning.

- All theoretical frameworks view the learner as an active contributor in the learning process.
- The entire context of learning is more important than any one variable alone. Learning is integrally related to the solution and understanding of real-life problems.
- Individuals' past experience and knowledge are critical in learning, in actions, and in acquiring new knowledge.
- Learners' values, attitudes and beliefs influence their learning and actions, and building learners' self awareness in this area is important for their development.
- Individuals as learners are capable of self-regulation, i.e., of setting goals, planning strategies, and evaluating their progress.
- The ability to reflect on one's practice (performance) is critical to lifelong, self-directed learning.

In another paper [2], I outlined five theories and their application to practice: andragogy, self-directed learning, self-efficacy, constructivism, and reflective practice. I refer the reader who is interested in theory to that article, as this chapter will address three different theories: cognitive apprenticeship, multiple intelligences, , and conditions of learning. I will provide a brief overview of each of these theories and will discuss the implications for educational practice., including a specific example for each drawn from medical education.

COGNITIVE APPRENTICESHIP

Cognitive Apprenticeship is a theory that outlines a method aimed primarily at teaching the processes that experts use to manage complex tasks.[4] The focus of this learning, through a guided experience method, is on cognitive and metacognitive skills rather than on the physical skills or processes of traditional apprenticeships. In traditional apprenticeship training, experts make their processes of performing and learning visible to the apprentice (e.g., a master carpenter or a skilled surgeon). The goal of cognitive apprenticeship is to make the thinking processes of a learning activity visible to both the learners and the teacher. The teacher is then able to employ the methods of traditional apprenticeship, i.e., modeling, coaching, scaffolding, and fading to effectively guide learners.[5]

In a classroom or clinical setting, the teacher models his/her thinking process, e.g., clinical reasoning, by talking out loud while working through a situation or problem, before turning the task over to learners. The teacher then coaches and scaffolds learners' efforts, gradually fading as the learners become more proficient. Cognitive apprenticeship should result in learners' greater understanding of the material and avoids "inert knowledge," helping them to apply their knowledge and skills to real-life situations. By observing the processes by which an expert listener or reader thinks and practices these skills, learners can learn on their own more skillfully.

A full cognitive apprenticeship approach would require the teacher to use the following steps in applying the method. However, based on the context and learners' educational stage, only selected steps may be used.

Modeling -- the expert carries out a task so that the learner can observe and build a conceptual model of the processes that are required to accomplish the task.

Coaching – the expert observes learners while they carry out a task and offering hints, feedback, modeling, and reminders.

Articulation – the expert encourages l;earners to use various methods of articulating their knowledge, reasoning, or problem-solving processes.

Reflection - learners compare their own problem-solving processes with those of the expert or another learner.

Exploration - involves pushing learners into a mode of problem-solving on their own.. Asking them to do exploration is critical, if they are to learn how to frame questions or problems that are interesting and that they can solve [5]

EXAMPLE

This method is commonly used in clinical settings, especially at the bedside to discuss patient cases. It also is employed by some surgeons with their clinical clerks, interns and/or residents. However, its application in clinical PBL or especially in lectures could enhance the effectiveness of these methods..

MULTIPLE INTELLIGENCES

This theory of human intelligence, developed by psychologist Howard Gardner [6,7] , suggests that there are at least seven ways that people have of perceiving and understanding the world. Gardner labels each of these as a distinct "intelligence"–in other words, a set of skills allowing individuals to learn, perform and solve problems that they face. While Gardner recognizes that his list of intelligences may not be exhaustive, he identifies the following seven [6,7]:

Verbal-Linguistic– ability to use words and language

*Logical-Mathematical–*capacity for inductive and deductive thinking and reasoning, as well as the use of numbers and the recognition of abstract patterns

*Visual-Spatial–*ability to visualize objects and spatial dimensions, and create internal images and pictures

*Body-Kinesthetic–*wisdom of the body and the ability to control physical motion

*Musical-Rhythmic–*ability to recognize tonal patterns and sounds, as well as a sensitivity to rhythms and beats

*Interpersonal–*capacity for person-to-person communications and relationships

*Intrapersonal–*spiritual, inner states of being, self-reflection, and awareness

IMPLICATIONS FOR MEDICAL EDUCATION

Traditional medical education heavily favors the verbal and and logical-intelligences. According to Gardner's theory, a more balanced curriculum that incorporates the arts, self-awareness, communication, and physical activity would produce a better professional. Gardner advocates instructional methods that appeal to all the intelligences, such as role playing, musical performance, cooperative learning, reflection, visualization, and story telling. This theory calls for assessment methods that take into account the diversity of intelligences, as well as self-assessment tools that help learners understand their intelligences.

EXAMPLE

The domain of communication skills training provides a good example of the use of multiple intelligences. The principles of effective communication are first learned through lectures, readings, and demonstrations. This is followed by role-playing with peers, progressing to simulated patients, and finally real patients (with supervision). Some specialized areas of human relations such as *setting personal boundaries* have been taught through the use of drawing on large sheets of paper placed on the floor, and, using coloured markers. [8] Music can also be used as a device to assist with memorization of bodies of facts such as learners need to do in their anatomy course.

CONDITIONS OF LEARNING

This theory stipulates that there are several different types or levels of learning. The significance of these classifications is that each different type requires different types of instruction. Gagne [9,10] identifies five major categories of learning: verbal information, intellectual skills, cognitive strategies, motor skills and attitudes. Different internal and external conditions are necessary for each type of learning. For example, for cognitive strategies to be learned, there must be a chance to practice developing new solutions to problems; to learn attitudes, the learner must be exposed to a credible role model or persuasive arguments.

Gagne advocates that learning tasks for intellectual skills can be organized in a hierarchy according to complexity: stimulus recognition, response generation, procedure following, use of terminology, discriminations, concept formation, rule application, and problem solving. The primary significance of the hierarchy is to identify prerequisites that should be completed to facilitate learning at each level. Prerequisites are identified by doing a task analysis of a learning/training task. Learning hierarchies provide a basis for the sequencing of instruction.

In addition, the theory outlines nine instructional events and corresponding cognitive processes, called the *events of instruction* [11]:

1) gaining attention (reception)
2) informing learners of the objective (expectancy)
3) stimulating recall of prior learning (retrieval)
4) presenting the stimulus (selective perception)
5) providing learning guidance (semantic encoding)
6) eliciting performance (responding)
7) providing feedback (reinforcement)
8) assessing performance (retrieval)
9) enhancing retention and transfer (generalization).

These events should satisfy or provide the necessary conditions for learning and serve as the basis for designing instruction and selecting appropriate media [11].

Implications for Medical Education

Although Gagne's theory is dated, it is based on many years of research and writing by one of psychology's most brilliant contributors and still can offer valuable insights and guidance to medical education practioners. His contributions are much too enormous to discuss here, so I am focusing on his events of instruction as these provide concrete steps for teaching. By following these steps, medical teachers can greatly improve their lectures, demonstrations, and one-on-one instruction in the clinical setting.

Example

The following example illustrates a teaching sequence for a first year medical student corresponding to the nine instructional events for the specific objective.

Objective: Recognize a hairline fracture of the fibula in an x-ray

1. Gain attention - show a variety of x-rays of normal and fractured fibulas
2. Identify objective - clarify objective: "What is a fibula? What is a hairline fracture?
3. Recall prior learning - review key points about the fibula and hairline fractures
4. Present stimulus – show a few x-rays of varous hairline fractures in a fibula
5. Guide learning- explain what to look for in the x-rays

6. Elicit performance - ask learners to identify a hairline fracture in the fibula in various rays, some having no fracture
7. Provide feedback – provide feedback re correct/incorrect responses and explain incorrect responses
8. Assess performance- provide scores or qualitative assessment, and remediation if needed
9. Enhance retention and transfer - show x-rays of different kinds of fibula fractures, including unusual hairline fractures, and discuss differences and similarities with learners

CONCLUSION

Although most educational theories have not been subjected to the rigours of randomized clinical (or educational) trials, they are based on logic, experience and best practices. Rather than debating the legitimacy of educational theory, I am urging medical educators to use theory as a guide to their practice and also as a validation of the excellent practices already carried out by exemplary teachers. There is also a debate among educators about whether these are actually theories, and there is some support for this view. However, whether we call these theories, models, or conceptual frameworks, I have argued here and elsewhere that they can provide excellent guidance for medical educators and also can evolve through being informed by effective practice. For the interested reader, the earlier monograph [1] and earlier paper [2] by this author, combined with this chapter, outline 16 educational theories that can be helpful to medical educators in their medical education practices.

REFERENCES

[1] *Kaufman*, DM and *Mann*, KV. Teaching and learning in medical education: How t*heory* can inform practice (2nd ed.) London, England: Association for the Study of Medical Education (ASME); 2007.

[2] Kaufman DM. Applying educational theory in practice. ABC of learning and teaching in medicine. British Medical Journal. 2003; 326: 213-16.

[3] Knowles MS, Associates. Andragogy in action: Applying modern principles of adult learning. San Francisco (CA): Jossey-Bass; 1984.

[4] Collins, A, Brown, JS, and Holum A. Cognitive apprenticeship: Making thinking visible. American Educator. 1991; 6 (11): 38-46.

[5] Aziz Ghefaili. Cognitive apprenticeship, technology, and the contextualization of learning environments. Journal of educational computing design and online learning. 2003; 4(Fall). [online] http://coe.ksu.edu/jecdt/vol_4/Articles/Aziz.htm.

[6] Gardner, H. Frames of Mind: The theory of multiple intelligences. New York: Basic Books; 1993.

[7] Gardner, H. Intelligence Reframed. Multiple intelligences for the 21st century. New York: Basic Books; 1999.

[8] Laidlaw T (2000) Setting Personal Boundaries. Workshops presented at Dalhousie University. Halifax, NS; 2000.
[9] Gagne, RM. The Conditions of Learning (4th ed.). New York: Holt, Rinehart and Winston; 1985.
[10] Gagne RM and Driscoll M, (1988). Essentials of learning for instruction. New Jersey: Prentice-Hall; 1988.
[11] Gagne RM, Briggs LJ, Wager WW. Principles of Instructional Design, 4th ed. Fort Worth, TX: Harcourt Brace Jovanovich College Publishers; 1992.

DAVID KAUFMAN, M.ENG., ED.D.

David Kaufman has been a faculty member at Concordia, Simon Fraser, Saint Mary's, and Dalhousie Universities, in the fields of Engineering, Computer Science, and Education. He has served as Director of Course Design for the Open Learning Agency (British Columbia's distance education institution), and Professor and Director of the Medical Education Unit in Dalhousie's Faculty of Medicine. He is the 1998 recipient of Dalhousie University's Instructional Leadership Award. Dr. Kaufman has presented more than 200 lectures and workshops at universities in North America, Europe, Asia and South America. He has published extensively with approximately 100 published articles and a co-authored book (*Distance Education in Canada, 1986)* to his credit. He also has been a reviewer for many journals, professional associations, and research granting councils. He has received numerous grants and contracts over the years. From 2001 to 2008, he served as Director, Learning and Instructional Development Centre at Simon Fraser University and Professor in the Faculty of Education. He was awarded a Social Sciences and Humanities Research Council of Canada (SSHRC) research grant of $3 million from 2003-08 to study the application of simulations and games for learning. He is currently a Professor in the Faculty of Education at SFU and Adjunct Professor in the Faculty of Medicine at the University of British Columbia.

In: New Research in Education Adult, Medical and Vocational ISBN 978-1-60741-873-3
Editors: Edmondo Balistrieri and Giustino DeNino © 2009 Nova Science Publishers, Inc.

Chapter 10

TEACHING MEDICAL STUDENTS ABOUT DECISION MAKING

Dylan Evans
School of Medicine, University College Cork, Ireland

ABSTRACT

Medical schools should devote more time and energy to helping medical students improve their decision making skills. Such instruction should include, at a minimum, an introduction to the theory of rational choice, an outline of the empirical research on human irrationality, and familiarisation with some of the tools and techniques that have been developed to help people to behave more rationally, such as decision-support systems and cognitive forcing strategies. The first and most important means for helping medical students to make more rational decisions is to introduce them to the research on cognitive biases, and to encourage them to analyse their own behaviour in the light of this research.

1. INTRODUCTION

The importance of including decision making in the medical curriculum is increasingly recognised by experts in medical education. The Scottish Deans' Medical Curriculum Group, for example, has stated that:

Decision making, and clinical reasoning and judgement are activities in which medical undergraduates should be proficient. The new medical graduate must continue to display such skills with the additional burden of increasing responsibility for their decisions and actions. This is undoubtedly one of the most stressful aspects of the transition between undergraduate and PRHO and therefore the achievement of these outcomes to a high standard is essential. [1]

Yet here the gap between theory and practice is perhaps greater than in any other area in medical education. If one were to allocate teaching time in proportion to the number of relevant learning outcomes listed in the report of The Scottish Deans' Medical Curriculum

Group, for example, about ten per cent of the medical curriculum should be devoted to the teaching of decision making skills, clinical reasoning, and judgement. Even the most forward-thinking of medical schools today fall far short of that lofty ambition. Some might question whether that should even be a goal at all. One aim of this chapter is to persuade such sceptics to reconsider their views on this matter.

This chapter is structured as follows. In the next section, I provide a brief outline of the study of rational decision making in order that those who are unfamiliar with this topic may gain a broad overview of the learning outcomes that should be included under this heading in the medical curriculum. In the following section, I review best practice in this area and discuss some practical suggestions on how instruction in decision making can be incorporated in the medical curriculum. I conclude with some brief remarks about the importance of considering rational decision making at the institutional level as well as at the individual one.

2. The Study of Rational Decision Making

The study of rational decision making has three elements:

1. *A normative element*: the theory of rational choice
2. *A descriptive element*: empirical research on human irrationality
3. *A prescriptive element*: tools and techniques for helping people to be more rational – i.e. for closing the gap between (1) and (2).

On the normative level, the theory of rational choice provides an account of what it means to make rational decisions. The basic idea is that a person makes a rational choice when he selects the alternative that maximises his expected utility [2]. The various alternatives that one may select are often expressed as a set, for example a set of j exhaustive and exclusive actions:

$$A = \{a_1,\ldots,a_i,\ldots a_j\}$$

For example, if a doctor must decide whether to prescribe antiobiotics, a placebo, or nothing, the set of alternatives is:

$$A = \{antibiotics,\ placebo,\ nothing\}$$

Once all the alternatives been identified, the decision-maker must calculate the expected utility of each. Expected utility is a measure that combines an estimate of how much good each alternative would produce if it worked, with an estimate of how likely it is that the alternative will, in fact, work. For a choice to be rational, the decision maker must choose the alternative with the highest expected utility.

Several decades of empirical research on how people actually make decisions have revealed that human behaviour departs significantly from the model of ideally rational behaviour described by the theory of rational choice. Moreover, it does so in certain systematic ways. In other words, human beings are not only irrational; they are also "predictably irrational" [3].

The systematic ways in which people make irrational choices are often attributed to a well-documented set of cognitive biases which skew human judgement in certain directions. For example, people tend to recall past events as being predictable even when they were not (hindsight bias), over-emphasize personality-based explanations for behaviours observed in others while under-emphasizing the role and power of situational influences on the same behaviour (fundamental attribution error), search for or interpret information in a way that confirms their preconception (confirmation bias), and claim more responsibility for successes than failures (self-serving bias). Many other cognitive biases have been identified by psychologists [4].

These biases are persistent and hard to overcome. Yet some progress has been made in devising mental techniques and tools that people can use to overcome or at least reduce bias and thereby make more rational decisions. These debiasing strategies include meta-cognition, instruction in rational choice theory and probability, decision-support systems, and cognitive forcing [5].

Meta-cognition, or "thinking about thinking", involves the ability to identify sources of irrationality in oneself and in others. As with any problem, one cannot even begin to overcome one's own cognitive biases if one is not even aware that they exist. Thus the first and most important means for helping people to behave more rationally is to make them familiar with the research on cognitive biases and human irrationality, and to encourage them to analyse their own behaviour in the light of this research.

Instruction in rational choice theory and probability tends to be reserved exclusively for students of economics and mathematics, but there is a strong case for making these subjects obligatory for students in all disciplines, and an overwhelming case for making them a central part of the medical curriculum. The most important medical instrument that a doctor will ever use is his own brain, and rational choice theory is the user's manual for this brilliant but unwieldy organ.

Decision-support systems include algorithms, guidelines, decision-rules, and computer-based decision aids. A large body of research has provided overwhelming evidence that clinicians who base their decisions on such decision aids make much better choices than those who disregard them and rely entirely on their clinical intuition [6]. However, many clinicians are still reluctant to use such decision-support systems, preferring to "use their heads instead of formulas" [7]. In order to overcome this tendency to disregard decision-support systems even when they are available, medical students should be taught to use various "cognitive forcing strategies" [8]. For example, they could be taught to always force themselves to consider a second diagnosis even when there seems to be an incontrovertible case for the initial diagnosis.

3. Incorporating Decision Making in the Medical Curriculum

As has already been noted, most medical schools devote far too little of their curricula to the content described in the previous section. Even when there is the will devote more time to such matters, there is often confusion about how best to go about this. In this section, therefore, I describe some ways in which the study of decision making can be incorporated more fully into the medical curriculum.

First, one must not neglect the traditional method for imparting information – the lecture. Lectures on expected utility theory, and on the empirical research on human irrationality, must be considered an essential component of the medical curriculum. Of course, these should be illustrated, wherever possible, by practical examples drawn from clinical practice. Unfortunately, there are plenty of examples of irrational behaviour in medicine, so the lecturer will not be at a loss here.

Secondly, students should be encouraged to apply the theory of expected utility to their own behaviour and to identify examples of irrationality in their own lives. Reflective learning logs are a suitable vehicle for such introspection, as are blogs, discussion groups, and private diaries.

Third, students should be introduced to a wide variety of decision-support systems, and given practical training in at least a few of these. In particular, they should be familiarised with a variety of clinical decision rules, and should know where to obtain information about such rules and how to evaluate them [9]. Seminars for discussion, and clinical skills workshops, would seem to be the most appropriate vehicles for this content. Along with this, students should be introduced in lectures and seminars to the literature that compares the effectiveness of unaided clinical judgement with the effectiveness of clinical judgement that is aided by decision support systems [6], and they should be taught to use cognitive forcing strategies.

An example of good practice in this area is the course entitled "Introduction to Medical Decision Making that is taught by Professor Goutham Rao at the School of Medicine in the University of Pittsburgh. This course provides an introduction to tools of analysis of particular relevance in clinical work and in the reading of medical literature. The goals of the course are to give students a foundation for using the basic and clinical sciences in medical decision making and to teach students to think critically about concepts relevant to medical decision making, including diagnostic reasoning, biostatistics and experimental design, etiology, prognosis and survival, therapies and studies of their effectiveness. The educational methods include lectures, small-group learning sessions, and writing and presenting a self-directed research paper. However, even this course falls somewhat short of the recommendations proposed here, as it does not appear to include any explicit instruction in expected utility theory.

4. Conclusion

Medical schools should devote more time and energy than is currently normal to helping medical students improve their decision making skills. Such instruction should include, at a minimum, an introduction to the theory of rational choice, an outline of the empirical research on human irrationality, and familiarisation with some of the tools and techniques that have been developed to help people to behave more rationally.

It is not often appreciated that the theory of rational choice applies equally to decisions made by organisations, institutions, and governments as it does to decisions made by individuals. A well-rounded course on medical decision making should therefore address role of incentive structures facing clinicians and health care managers in generating optimal health outcomes, and should help individual clinicians to understand the economic implications of their clinical decisions. Medical students should, therefore, be able to apply rational choice theory to the analysis of public health policies, and to discuss how we might, as a society, arbitrate between conflicting agendas of healthcare resource allocation (rationing). This may be a utopian goal, but it is surely one worth striving for.

REFERENCES

[1] The Scottish Deans' Medical Curriculum Group. Learning Outcomes for the Medical Undergraduate in Scotland: A foundation for competent and reflective practitioners; 2000.

[2] Neumann Jv, Morgenstern O. Theory of Games and Economic Behavior. 2007 ed. Princeton: Princeton University Press 1944.

[3] Ariely D. Predictably Irrational: The Hidden Forces That Shape Our Decisions London: HarperCollins 2008.

[4] Kahneman D, Slovic P, Tversky A. Judgement Under Uncertainty: Heuristics and Biases. Cambridge: Cambridge University Press 1982.

[5] Bradley CP. Can we avoid bias? British Medical Journal. 2005;330:784.

[6] Dawes RM, Faust D, Meehl PE. Clinical versus actuarial judgement. Science. 1989;243:1668-74.

[7] Kleinmuntz B. Why we still use our heads instead of formulas: toward an integrative approach. Psychological Bulletin. 1990;107(3):296-310.

[8] Crosskerry P. The importance of cognitive errors in diagnosis and strategies to minimise them. Academic Medicine. 2003;78:775-80.

[9] Purcell GP. What makes a good clinical decision support system. British Medical Journal. 2005;330:740-41.

INDEX

B

C

H

I

N

O

P

Q

R

S

T

U

V